10,000 years of Weight Watching: The Surprising History of Dieting.

TABLE OF CONTENTS

Introduction

The year is 2015 and we are in the midst of what the media and authorities are claiming to be "An Obesity Epidemic." There are many reasons and opinions about why this is so, or even if there really is an epidemic. The truth is, we have gone so far away from nature that human beings are suffering from diseases such as obesity and Type 2 Diabetes in epidemic proportions.

The reason I have written this book is that I have realised, through research and study, that our fascination with body shape is nothing new. To be a certain weight or shape has always been a focus of our attention. In the days of the hunter/gatherer, it was desired that the body was able to conserve fat, simply because the fear of famine. Being plump was also considered a good point in favour of a woman's fertility. Just like bears eat and preserve fat for the winter months of hibernation, so humans have had to do that, too, throughout the course of history.

The problem these days, at least in the Western world, and increasingly in most parts of modern society, is that there is never a time when we are short of food. But evolution has not caught up with that idea. Consequently, our fat reserves are never burnt up.

We begin with examining the ancient ways of seeing the body and the desire to be either thin or fat. We'll also look at ancient civilisations to see what they ate, from the early Egyptians to the 18th Century.

As we approach the 19th and 20th centuries, we will see that people were becoming ever more desperate to be able to eat and remain thin, and what they did about it.

I have broken the 20th Century down into decades, so that the reader can clearly see the developments that led to where we are today. I hope that by reading this book, people will come to realise that the battle with body shape is nothing new. People who are constantly watching their weight and, in some cases, losing the battle to keep it under control, can feel isolated and think that they are to blame.

But I have also endeavoured to point out that during the mid- 20th century we started to lose control over what we were eating.

In the last chapter, however, I have shown that the tables are turning. Thanks to modern technological information, the weight watcher can now take back a certain amount of control and the battle is not lost.

We no longer have to be in the hands of the authorities, but can find out for ourselves how we can eat well and accept ourselves for what we are.

Despite the fact that we feel we have to diet, we do not have to be stick thin to be healthy. We can make the right choices without restrictive dieting.

Chapter 1. How We Moved From Being Hunter/Gatherers.

We can start to look at diet all the way back to about 9000 B.C. Previous to that time, we had been hunter gatherers, living on meat by hunting and gathering leaves, fruit, berries, vegetables and nuts.

Imagine that you are living in a cave, and that you and the family need food. The woman of the cave, along with her women friends, are just seeing their mates off for the next hunt. The men are off to find the meat or fish of the day or week.

Meanwhile the women of the tribe or community will go and gather wild berries, roots, fruits, nuts, seeds, and leaves or herbs.

The men would come back with the meat and fish, probably already skinned as soon as they caught it. By now the women have lit a fire ready to cook, and will have prepared the vegetables. (We are assuming that fire has been discovered)

We know all this because of the work of palaeontologists and archaeologists who have put the picture together from digs and discoveries. We also know that there was very little of the modern diseases such as arthritis, cancer, etc., because of research done by scanning bones and other means.

It is noticeable that finds of female statuettes from these times were rounded and full bellied. There is controversy over the significance of the shape of these statuettes and whether they signified the desired or ideal shape or the actual shape of women. Was this a shape that was aspired to as a sign of health and fertility? Was it just a symbol of fertility?

Then, about 10,000 years ago, a revolution came about with the way we ate, with the onset of the age of agriculture. People had realised that they did not need to be hunting miles away from home, and that they could enclose the animals in pens; breed them, rear them and eat them. The change developed over the next few thousand years and did not happen overnight.

Whether it was for the better is a worthwhile study. According to Juliann Schaeffer of "Today's Dietician" (link below) we can learn a lot about how the body has not evolved as fast as the ways in which our diet has changed since this time.

Before the Age of Agriculture, our diet did not contain milk after a young age or of course any of milk's derivatives. Many people today cannot digest lactose in milk, which is the sugar.

Illnesses such as eczema, rheumatoid arthritis and psoriasis, which are a relatively common and modern phenomenon, have been shown to improve once dairy products have been left out of the diet, for example.

There are claims that the diseases which abound in modern society such as cardiovascular, cancer, diabetes and obesity are due to our genes not keeping up with progress.

Loren Cordain, PhD, a professor and author of *The Paleo Diet*, says: "Although a number of genetic changes have occurred since the agricultural revolution, the majority of the human genome has resulted from the environment of our hunter-gatherer ancestors and earlier."

Cordain goes on to say that previous to the agricultural revolution, humans had been evolving for millions of years, but since then, there have only been 330 human generations. From this we can see that our bodies have simply not had time to get used to the rapid change in what we eat.

Nevertheless, humans found that we could grow wheat, barley, peas, lentils and other grains in enclosed "fields", by digging up the land and planting seeds. Ploughing did not start until around 4000 BC, when horses and donkeys began to be domesticated.

By 7000 BC we were domesticating sheep, pigs and goats, and a thousand years later, cattle too.

Farming first began in what is known today as the middle-east, around the area of Israel to Southeast Turkey and then spread to Europe.

In Egypt the Nile was already being used for irrigation. When it flooded every year, and dried back, it made for very fertile land.

The Egyptians are one of the first groups of people to use agriculture as a means of building wealth. They farmed staple food crops, such as barley and wheat, and of course are known for their ingenuity with flax and papyrus, using papyrus for documentation.

As well as certain kinds of meat and fish, they consumed foods such as grains, vegetables, pulses, beans, lentils, onions, garlic, lettuce and parsley. Fruits included carob, olive, apple and pomegranate. Peaches and pears are also mentioned, not to forget the palm date.

It was the Celts in France and Ireland who thought of the idea of fields, thus dividing up the land in a fair and equal manner. The Celts also started brewing beer from barley. They raised cattle and other livestock for use in milking and slaughtering for food. Thus, the need for hunting in the wild was not so essential in European civilisation.

In China, farming began about 5000 BC, where the primary crops were rice and millet. Dogs and pigs were also domesticated, followed by horses. The dogs and horses were not always to eat, but to live among people for their use.

Having to watch our weight seems to have been around for a very long time. There is a myth among people who study and suffer from bulimia that the Romans had special vomitoriums for people to throw up the food that they had eaten at feasts, to make room for more food, and to keep their weight down. But that is all it is; a myth.

There were vomitoriums, but they were not used for vomiting. They were passageways below or behind a row of seats in an amphitheatre or stadium, for people to exit quickly at the end of a performance. Vomitaria is plural for vomitorium and the two Latin words combined (vomo, vomere) meaning to 'spew forth'. So it was a way for the crowds to spew forth from the theatres.

Nevertheless, the Romans did apparently eat and purge several times a day. On the constant lookout for a slimmer physique, dieters have always gone to extreme lengths. In Roman times the upper class men did indeed like their wives and daughters to be slim.

Just as in modern times, they looked for quick fixes and did not seem willing to find a way that would make them lose weight and keep it off, and what is more, to stay healthy. In other words, change their lifestyle and change the way that they think. Looking back through the ages, we shall see that this is nothing new.

In an interesting article on this subject Mind Hacks (reference below) tells of a letter to the *Journal of the American Academy of Child and Adolescent Psychiatry* in which the authors talk of evidence from ancient Rome showing that the culture of thinness was nothing new.

In the account of an ancient comedy a young man declares his love for a 16-year old girl who seems to look different, and he protests against the contemporary emphasis on thinness.

He talks of mothers who strive to make the girls have sloped shoulders and a squeezed chest so that they look slim. He goes on to describe the girl he loves who has unusual looks with: "A natural complexion, a plump and firm body, full of vitality"

Looking at a normal way of eating for those days, it seems that the Romans had breakfast at dawn, followed at around 11 a.m. with a small lunch. In the evening, they had what was called *Cena*. When the Greeks came along, this was changed slightly to an increase of the amount of food in the evening and *Cena* was consumed in the afternoon, followed by a light supper.

This routine was also followed by the lower strata of society because it fit in with work routines.

Flat round loaves of bread made from emmer, which is a grain related to wheat, with a little added salt was eaten and this was sometimes dipped into wine and eaten with cheese and olives.

Milk, fruit, eggs, wild boar, beef, pork, lamb, duck, goose, chickens, fish and shellfish were included in the diet, but usually as a luxury and not every day.

Sausages were first mentioned at these times too. A light-hearted reference taken from the link below says that they were made from blood, leeks and onion, and yolks of hard boiled eggs. Brains were sometimes used, or wheat along with chopped meat and pepper.

The sausages were a convenient way for Roman soldiers to carry their food with them.

There was also a kind of porridge made from emmer, water, salt and fat. Olive oil being the choice for the upper classes.

Fruit was eaten in season: apples, pears, quinces, pomegranates and figs, and later on, oranges too.

Vegetables included cabbage, lettuce, endive, onion, leeks, radishes, turnips and cucumber. This was the time when carrots were purple; they were not changed in colour for many centuries.

Fish was more common than meat, as it was easier to catch and cook. Oyster farming had already started, too.

Wine was high in alcohol, so was usually drunk with water. So this practice is not new to the 21st century, even though they did not have to worry about drinking and driving. Beer was considered vulgar and not consumed by the upper classes.

The Greek diet was quite similar and they also had pancakes. *Maza* was also eaten, which you can still find in authentic Greek restaurants today. I can remember having them dished up to us at a drinks party held my some Greek friends here in the UK and they were delicious.

Cereals such as wheat and barley were around. Wheat grains were softened and made into gruel. Also served were the same fruits and vegetables the Romans ate.

How much fish and meat you ate varied in accordance to your wealth and location, just as with the Romans. Also dairy foods, though these would usually come from goats and sheep, rather than cattle.

An interesting fact from around this time is that we can apparently attribute the discovery of using yeast in bread to the Egyptians at around 4000 B.C. Sugar was first produced in India around 3000 B.C.

The conclusion one comes to in reading the history of diet in general, up until the Middle Ages, is that it was very similar in all regions of the world. A basic diet of grains, fruit, berries, nuts, seeds, vegetables, meat, fish and birds. Considering of course that people were living on the land and not removed from it as much as we are today.

Moving on to the Middle Ages from around 400 to 1400 A.D., farming started to improve. Most people, including the peasants, owned an ox, so they used to team up oxen from other families, to pull the plough.

By now in addition to cattle, pigs, sheep and goats, there is talk of keeping chickens, which were used for eggs and eating just as they are today.

Meat was preserved throughout the winter by salting, and the same with fish.

According to Local Histories, (link below) the rich ate well in that period. Their diet consisted of beef, mutton, pork, venison and a variety of birds. It seems that the church imposed an intermittent fasting diet even then, as they declared that Wednesday, Friday and Saturday were fast days when people were not allowed to eat meat.

Poor people, on the other hand, had a monotonous diet of coarse, dark bread and cheese. If they were lucky, they would have a rabbit or even some pork. The evening meal was something like gruel which consisted of grains which had been soaked and then mixed with hot water. Maybe some vegetables, and on rare occasions the before-mentioned rabbit or pork. Nuts, vegetables and fruit were eaten in season.

8

This would have lasted up until the 16th century, and the Elizabethan age. At this time, vegetables were considered food to be eaten by the poor. The rich ate meat and fish which consisted of salmon, eel, venison, beef, lamb and fowl, which in our modern day is chicken. In those days you ate fowl, which was an older bird.

Their dessert would have consisted of a variety of pastries, cakes and crystallised fruit, usually referred to as sweetmeats.

Bread was considered a staple of the Elizabethan diet. The type of bread depended on whether you were rich or poor. The rich ate white bread. Perhaps this was the reason why we turned to white bread after the Second World War; the belief having been handed down through the generations that white bread was a luxury!

The diet for both the rich and poor lacked fruit and vegetables. There was a lot of scurvy around for that reason, due to a lack of vitamin C.

For a time, food and diet remained much the same in the Eastern hemisphere, throughout Europe and the Far East; the only change was that tomatoes and potatoes were added during the 17th century.

In the 17th century, something called chop houses were introduced where people met to eat meat.

Although the fork had been used in more ancient times, it was re-introduced as an eating utensil around this same time.

With progress, many new foods were introduced, but as in previous times only the rich benefitted from them. In the UK, these new foods included bananas and pineapples.

Starbucks and Costa were not the first to start coffee bars, because the 17th Century saw coffee arrive in Britain and brought about what were known as coffee houses.

The rest of the diet remained the same as in the 16th century

In the 18th century, the food and diet in England seemed to deteriorate, due to increasing population and difficulties with transport.

As well as the meats consumed in the previous centuries, venison became a status symbol. Probably because among the rich this was a meat that was hunted and shot for a hobby, as opposed to hunting for necessity as in the days of the hunter gatherers.)

I was amused when recently I came across an article in a newspaper entitled, "Would You Eat a Reindeer?" The writer seemed to be ignorant of the fact that reindeer are venison and we have been eating that for centuries!

Meat seems to have been the mainstay of peoples' diets, as they were suspicious of fruits and vegetables, thinking that they would give them indigestion or even the plague. One reason for this was because they were covered in mud and the vendors used to lick them clean with their tongues!

However, this was also the century when sailors were dying of scurvy when they were at sea for any great length of time. This came to the attention of the Admiralty who realised that this was because of the need for citrus fruits. They would not have known it was related to the lack of Vitamin C, as vitamins were not discovered until the early 1900's. But they certainly saw the connection. An early example of connecting up cause and effect.

Cheese also became more popular and the English developed their now famous cheddar.

The average consumption of sugar was about 4 kilograms a year. (As opposed to our present consumption of 35 kilos)

The Colonial diet was somewhat richer and better, because the land was not so crowded and there were cleaner conditions. The average New Englander had a simple diet, and the English settlers tended to stick to their old ways of eating.

Meanwhile, in other parts of America, it seems that the cultivation of crops begins in the Tehuacan Valley, southeast of present-day Mexico City.

Because we do not have a written history of America, we are relying more on archaeology to tell us what was going on.

According to a report in May 1997 in the journal *Science* by Bruce D Smith, an assessment was based on the discovery of the remains of seeds, rinds and stems in a cave named Guila Naquitz near Oaxaca, in Mexico. This indicated that squash was the first New World crop and that agriculture developed in the New World around the same time that it did in the Near East and Asia.

It is reckoned in the same report that agriculture was more difficult to evolve in the New World than it was in the Near East and Mesopotamia, where it was easier to cultivate the fields.

However, in Mexico it seems that there was a reverse situation, according to archaeologist Kent Flannery. He says that the first villages don't show up until around 1500 B.C.

According to Flannery, by 2500 B.C. there were true farmers around who were raising beans, corn and squash.

People in America did not settle so quickly in permanent villages and they lived on woodland deer, rabbits, turtles and birds. And of course, buffalo were hunted quite early on in history.

In America at this time the Aztecs grew tomatoes, avocados, beans, peppers, pumpkins, peanuts and amaranth seeds. They also ate fruit, rabbits, dogs, turkeys and armadillos. So you could say that their diet was different! Their staple food was maize.

The Inca ate a similar diet, plus potatoes and quinoa.

The Maya were pretty busy slashing and burning in agriculture. So although it would not have been on the scale of today's destruction of the Amazon forest, it is nothing new. As one area lost its fertility, so they would slash and burn another to prepare for planting.

Their staple foods were maize, sweet potatoes and squashes. Interestingly, they also kept bees for honey.

So we can see then that there was not really a lot of difference between each known area of the world. And food and diet remained the same for centuries, with the growth of grains getting bigger all the time.

It is notable however, that all through history; it is only the better off that needed to be worried about their weight and dieting. In the next chapter, we'll start to look at the change in attitude at the turn of the 20th century and how it came about.

References.

http://www.historyworld.net.

http://www.todaysdietitian.com/newarchives/040609p36.shtml

http://factsanddetails.com

http://www.sausageobsession.com/history_of_sausage/

http://en.wikipedia.org/wiki/Ancient_Egyptian_agriculture

http://mindhacks.com/2009/10/22/size-zero-culture-in-ancient-rome/

http://www.localhistories.org/middle.html

http://en.wikipedia.org/wiki/Health_and_diet_in_Elizabethan_England

Chapter 2. The 1800's: Attitude Begins to Change.

Although food itself did not change in the industrial era, which began in the 1800's, it did mark the beginning of what we call "fad dieting." What exactly is a fad diet?

According to the medical dictionary found here; http://medical-dictionary.thefreedictionary.com/fad+diet

This is one definition of fad-diet.

"Any number of weight-reduction diets that either eliminate one or more of the essential food groups, or recommend consumption of one type of food in excess, at the expense of other foods. Fad diets rarely follow sound nutritional principles for weight loss, which focus on ingesting fewer calories and/or consuming more energy through exercise; fad diets are generally not endorsed by the medical profession."

However, here http://dictionary.reference.com/browse/fad

The dictionary breaks it down into 2 definitions and separates the meaning of the two words.

Noun.

1. An intense but short lived fashion; craze.

2. A personal idiosyncrasy or whim.

And the word diet simply means a way of eating. But in this context the whole has been made into one by the medical dictionary's definition. For the purposes of this chapter, I am using the second definition.

I have added more about the first definition elsewhere in this book.

We already know watching weight or size was nothing new, and we have already seen that the Romans liked their women to be slim and shapely.

Yet the Industrial era seems to coincide with what I can find on the history of fad diets.

But first a look at the staple diet around that time.

As far as food was concerned, it seems that living in the countryside was a lot healthier, providing that you were not in an area plagued by poor harvests and crop disease. As the urban districts got grimier and more crowded, it became more difficult to obtain good, fresh food.

As the century wore on however, things began to improve with better transport from railways. For many, foods such as dairy produce, meat and fish appeared for the first time. Much like today with tropical fruits appearing on our tables due to better transport between countries.

Whilst the factory worker gulped down his cup of black tea and hunky slice of dry bread, however, the better off were enjoying tea served with milk and dainty cakes.

Eggs, bread, potatoes, rice, flour, vegetables and cheese, were what the poorest families were eating. Foods such as meats and fish were the fare of the better off.

So it makes you wonder why people would have needed to diet. Nevertheless, they did!

It seems that fad diets were being used in the 19th century. And just like today, people were going to extreme measures to lose weight.

According to historian and author Louise Foxcroft *"Dieting back then was about all-round mental and physical health. People really got a taste for fad dieting in the 19th Century. It is during this time that things tip over into dieting more for aesthetic reasons and the diet industry explodes."*

It was also in the 19th century that "Fletcherism" was investigated and used. Horace Fletcher was an art dealer who had weight problems and lost 40 lbs from this method. His diet required that you could eat anything you liked, but you needed to chew each piece of food 32 times, until it was liquid in your mouth, before swallowing it.

His theory was that people were not chewing their food enough and that for ideal health we should chew our food until it is liquid to absorb the nutrients.

I once saw this done in an experiment on TV and it was quite successful, but very difficult to do

Also, and perhaps more sensibly, Fletcher taught that we should not eat until we are really hungry.

That way, we will eat a lot less, won't be overweight or obese, and we will save a lot of money on food. But not much in time!

Fletcherism became a part of the American psyche at this period, but I imagine that the working classes would have been too busy to practice this.

According to Dr. Louise Foxcroft, author of *Calories and Corsets*, diet pills also became popular. Some were arsenic and other poisons and became increasingly big business. Along with arsenic, strychnine was also used. They were advertised as speeding up the metabolism, much like amphetamines do, which we shall read about when we come to the 1950's.

Vinegar, or cider vinegar was suggested as a diet aid, and is still recommended 100 years later.

During this era, we find the first celebrity to be observed by the public to be struggling with weight issues was the famous poet Lord Byron.

According to Foxcroft, he was 5ft 8.5 which was quite tall for those days, and his weight fluctuated between 9.5 stone and 14. So it seems that he was what subsequently became known as a yo-yo dieter. Even though he was an active man, he struggled with weight issues.

Foxcroft goes on to say that he was a vegetarian most of the time, and often lived on dry biscuits and white wine for days, then occasionally he would eat large helpings of meat and desserts.

This is the typical pattern of bulimics and compulsive eaters of today. They go on very strict diets, virtually starve themselves, and then end up undoing all the work by bingeing.

Byron realised the harm he was doing but could not stop himself.

He also drank green tea; so nothing new there either.

He apparently used to drink a lot of vinegar and soaked his potatoes in the stuff. This resulted in diarrhoea and vomiting.

Because of his celebrity status, people found out about it and started worrying about their weight too, including Queen Victoria. This in turn led a semi-epidemic of starvation and hysteria now referred to as Victorian Anorexia, and was known as a way for women to keep the tiny waists that they aspired to have.

Does all this sound familiar somehow?

Another extreme way of losing weight was to use parasites, such as the tapeworm. Maria Callas was purported to use this one. But it has now been suggested that this, too, is a myth.

The tapeworm was swallowed in the form of a pill and the tapeworm would reach maturity in the intestines, thus absorbing all the goodness from food and, as with the vinegar diet, brought about diarrhoea, vomiting and of course, loss of weight.

Don't read on if you are squeamish!

When the desired weight was reached, the dieter then took an anti-parasitic pill to excrete the worm which could grow up to 9 metres in length. You can imagine the intestinal, rectal and digestive problems this could bring about.

The side effects were known to include headaches, eye problems, meningitis, epilepsy and dementia.

I have purposely taken a separate look at William Banting. People who are fans of the low carbohydrate way of eating would not count his diet as a fad. Banting was born in 1796 and died in 1878. Interestingly, he was a distant relative of Frederick Banting, who discovered insulin.

He is known to be the first to produce the low carbohydrate diet. Although his diet consisted of some carbohydrate, it was very little. He undertook this way of eating at the suggestion of Dr William Harvey after struggling to lose weight for some time. Harvey had been studying it in the context of diabetes management. Which is ironic as the debate about Type 2 diabetes and carbohydrate still continues to this day. (For more on this subject read Robert Ludwig's book *Fat Chance*)

In 1863, Banting wrote a booklet called *Letter on Corpulence, Addressed to the Public* containing the plan for the diet that he had followed and in which he successfully lost the weight that he had been struggling to lose for years.

It specified four meals a day, consisting of meat, green vegetables, fruits, and dry wine. He avoided sugar, saccharine, starch, beer, milk and butter. He had two slices of bread a day.

I am "Banting" became a popular way of saying that you were on a low-carbohydrate diet. So you see, Atkins was not the first to come onto the scene with this idea.

The modern take on this diet is of course the low-carbohydrate idea. As with Atkins, false rumours were spread about the diet destroying his health. But it influenced the modern day investigations into this way of eating.

I will add that today's low-carbohydrate diet would include butter, but milk does contain carbohydrate.

Gary Taubes discusses it in his book *Good Calories, Bad Calories.*

So now let's diverge for a moment and take a look at the History of Obesity, which is the reason we started dieting in the first place.

Firstly of course, the only criteria for judging a person's status in the size category would be how a person looks. Evidence of the first weighing scales to be found was around 2000 BC, but it is doubtful that weighing people would have been common. Bathroom scales were not in use until recent times. Even when I first started dieting, I had to go to the chemist, drug store or doctor's surgery.

Going further back, stone-age artifacts have shown that it may have even been desirable to be fat, as of course this would have stood people in good stead in times of famine.

So it looks as if obesity did exist in primitive and ancient societies. It has been discovered in skeletons from over 20,000 years ago. However, it was not frowned upon and if you were a woman, fat reflected favourably on your potential for fertility and pregnancy.

Looking at the link between what people ate and obesity, we can go back as far as ancient Egypt. Stone reliefs show a fat cook being presented to Ankh-MA-Hor. (Sixth Dynasty, 2310-2180 B.C.)

Studies of mummies have shown folds of skin, which suggested that they were fat. But though plump people were not uncommon in ancient Egypt, it was not the ideal shape. They, too, liked their women to be slender.

The goddesses such as Venus and Diana were plump and matronly with round bodies. They were glorified as the Mother Earth image. However, the daughters and wives of Greeks were expected to be slim and beautiful in order to look seductive in revealing clothes. (Sound familiar?)

It was in classical times that it began to be recognised as a problem. Aristophanes, a fifth century B.C. Greek comedy writer described obese men as "Bloated, gross, and pre-seniled....they are fat rogues with big bellies and dropsical legs, whose toes by the gout are tormented."

The ancient Greek Hippocrates connected up the facts that sudden death was more common in obese people and that being obese caused other diseases.

It is said that he also realised the connection between energy in and energy out, although he would not have referred to calories as they are a scientific term in later centuries. There is some controversy with the calorie theory, which will be worth following up if you are interested, in the Gary Taube's book mentioned earlier, and there are numerous references to the subject on-line.

Even as far back as 500-400 B.C. Hindu physicians are credited with recognising the sugary taste of diabetic urine and that the disease was connected with overweight people who ate excessive sweet and sugary foods.

In ancient China, they were aware of the dangers of obesity, and how it affected longevity.

There is a more positive approach to obesity in cultures where there is scarcity and illness. In Africa some tribes plump up their women for child bearing. A slim bride will be plumped up because it is a sign of wealth and plenty.

In 1418 it was claimed that Queen Catalina died of a stroke, possibly caused by her "great size" and it is well known that Henry VIII suffered great ill health because of it. He was known as a warmonger and had a huge appetite for food as well as wives!

An interesting observation by the Dawn Centre, (which is a centre for eating disorders, and you can find them in the link below of the same name,) is that once the connection was made to illness and obesity in the 17th century, knowledge on how to reverse it was unclear.

My observation in turn is that the controversy is still going on over three hundred years later! The doctors at that time had no idea what was causing it, and they did not believe that what you ate had anything to do with it.

The Dawn Centre goes on to say that all through the 1800's the controversy continued, until the early 19th century, when Dr William Wadd, a physician of the English court, made the connection between overindulgence at the table and being fat. During the 17th and 18th century, being obese or overweight was seen as sinful, because it meant that you were committing the sin of gluttony.

Perhaps this explains why to this day many people feel guilty because they are overweight or obese; they have inherited this interpretation in some way.

In the Renaissance period, the artist Rubens is known for his paintings of obese females. But if you look at these paintings, the women cannot be classed as obese. Also bear in mind that art can be according to the artist's impression. Many people have referred to this period as a time when it was accepted for women to be bigger. But when you compare the size to what we consider our standards nowadays to what is considered obese, these women can be categorised as shapely, but not obese.

.

Moving on in time, during the 1930's and 40's, plump babies and children were seen as bonny and healthy. There used to be competitions for bonny babies, and the plump ones were seen as the bonniest.

Attitudes over the last 60 years have changed obesity into a something a bit easier to define and this book will look at that in greater depth.

We can see that being fat, obese or overweight, has always been frowned upon in western circles. Generally speaking, it seems to be caused by what people are eating and the amounts that they are eating. In the last 100 years or so though, there seems to be many ideas and theories about what works and what does not work.

As I mentioned earlier, there is now a lot of controversy going on about the calorie in must equal calorie out theory. But it is far more complicated than that.

However, the good news is that in the 21st century there are other ideas coming to the fore, including emotional and psychological differences and that everyone is as different in their nutritional needs as they are in everything else. There is no one diet that fits all.

How is obesity defined in 2015?

As well as being able to see the condition, it is also defined in various tables; the most well-known is the BMI table.

It is quite complicated to calculate as follows;

Divide your weight in kilograms by your height in metres.

Then divide the answer again to get your BMI

This way, you have to go by the tables as follows.

Under 18 you are too thin.

18 to 25 is the healthiest.

25 to 30 is overweight

Over 30 you are classed as obese. However the table below is by far the easiest to go by.

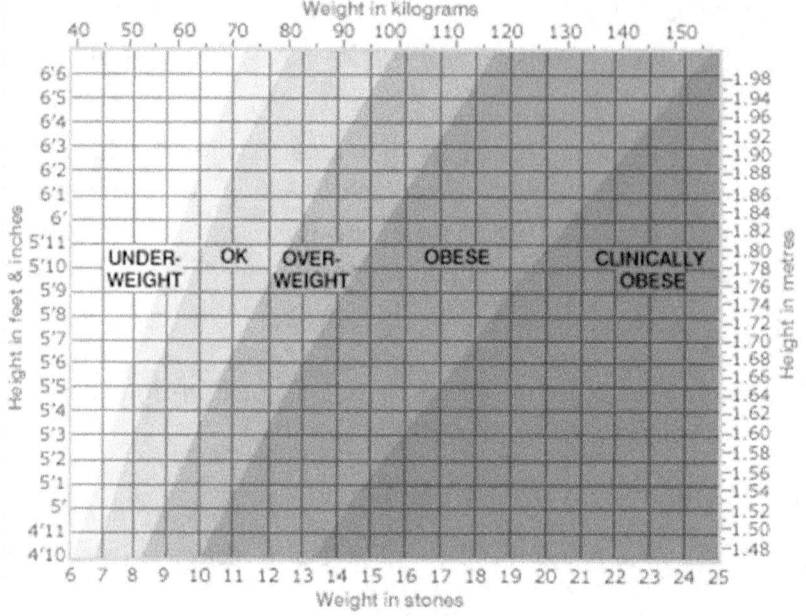

References.

http://www.dawn-centre.ie/index.php?page=Page&op=show&id=90

Chapter 3. Who Were the People Who Needed to Diet? 1900 to 1910

The twentieth century was to be a big turning point with the way that humans ate. At the start of the century, many poor children were suffering from malnutrition, with many of them sitting down to nothing more than a plate of potatoes and scraps of bread. It is ironic that 100 years later, there are people still suffering from malnutrition, but because the quality of the food that we are eating is so bad. People now have a choice, but are ignoring healthy foods and going for the empty, junk, fast, refined foods.

Food was very expensive in 1904 and a working class family spent about 44% of their income on food. But by the 1930's they only spent 35%. In the 1950's about 20%.

It is interesting to note that it is reckoned that now in the 2010's we only spend about 10% of our income on food and that is because we have other priorities. Although percentage wise it looks as if food is cheaper, in actuality it is not. We fill our homes with "stuff" consisting of technology, beautiful furniture, with carpets and sofas that need replacing quite often.

We feel we have to keep up with what is fashionable in the home rather than what is practical. Consequently, we do not put what we are eating at the top of the list of priorities as they would have in the early 20th century. In those days, the less well off made food a priority, but they also did not have all the necessary material items that we have to buy these days.

For example, because of our geographical positions many people have to have a car.

Computers are a necessity because more and more big firms are expecting you to have online accounts with them. Even some banks are closing down branches.

Because our shopping habits have changed, we have to have freezers and refrigerators.

There are not many homes without a television.

I recently had a discussion with someone about our expectations. A certain political party had put out a poster claiming that in the 1960's a man could keep his family comfortably and be the only bread winner. They were of course, saying that their party could do better, and it was the other party's fault. But I pointed out to her that the reason why a man could keep his family in the 60's was because that family's expectations were simpler. I was wasting my breath, as she could not see what I meant.

However, back to the subject at hand, around the turn of the 20th century, a typical breakfast would have been bread and butter, and a cup of tea. This seems to have been the standard fare even for the upper classes. Maybe at times a boiled egg to go with it.

Breakfast seems to be a meal that was taken at all sorts of times and was never a regular meal. When you break down the word breakfast that is exactly what it is, breaking your fast. It seems that it was only a small meal for the poor and the rich alike.

Kedgeree or a piece of fried bread with buttered eggs and bacon was also a popular breakfast for the better off.

Farmers used to get up in the very early hours of the morning and come in for their breakfast mid-morning. In fact, many of them still do this to this day.

So it seems that what to have for breakfast if you wanted to lose weight around this time was not really an issue. Having said that though, there was a book which made an appearance in 1904 called *The No Breakfast Diet Plan* and *The Fasting Cure* by Edward Hooker Dewey.

This book was written with several diseases of the body in mind, among them apoplexy, obesity and digestive disorders.

A quote from the book reads: *"Why is the hardest labour more easily performed and for more hours without a breakfast."*

There has always been a quandary over how to address the name of a meal. It seems that around this time, the first meal of the day was breakfast. The midday meal was lunch or luncheon, and then afternoon tea was at 5p.m. and dinner at 7.30 p.m.

However, the working class family with father coming home to the midday meal would address that meal as dinner and the evening meal as supper.

These meals would vary depending on which country you lived in. For example, in Germany you would have afternoon coffee and cake, whereas in the UK or America, the gentry and plantation owners in other countries would have tea and sandwiches and cake. Bearing in mind that the sandwiches were dainty quarter rounds with the crusts cut off and filled with nothing but cucumber. The cakes would be delicate and would only just be a small mouthful.

But the factory workers and schoolchildren would have been eating a big, hearty sandwich either for lunch or a snack.

The evening dinner would most often be an accompaniment to some sort of entertainment for the upper class, and would consist of game, fish or some cut of meat. Usually with a light soup, followed by a desert.

In a book written by a Mrs. Francis Carruthers in 1905 called *The Century Home Cook Book*, she says:

"Indeed, the hours for eating must be regulated by the hours of employment. If one is in the whirl of fashionable life of a great city, and nightly out until four or five o'clock in the morning, the heavy meal of the day must come later, and a light supper at midnight becomes a necessity."

"If you are a hard working farmer, living in the country and going to bed between nine and ten, the meal hours must correspond."

*"**Common Sense Hours**" – Meals should be timed by common sense. It is probably more healthful to take a rather light breakfast, which in a malarious country, should always include coffee. At noon, a more substantial meal is in order, but as, in this country (USA, my insertion) several hours of hard work are to follow, it should not be too heavy, and a quarter or half hour's rest after it is time well spent.*

The Dyspepsia so common in this country comes from taking, as a habit, more food than is necessary, and then working hard with head or body immediately afterwards. Digestion requires repose and most people eat far more than nature calls for.

The best time for a heavy dinner is after the hard work for the day is over and a couple or more hours can be given to comfortable rest, reading, conversation or light amusement.

Eat slowly, not too much at any one meal, take small pieces which can easily be masticated, and do not go directly from the table to violent exercise or severe brain work.

Make your dinner (or evening meal, by whatever name you choose to call it,) a pleasant, social affair, which tempts you to linger over it; not a place to bolt, in haste, a certain amount of unmasticated food, and then fly from.

Cultivate the beauties and the social aspects of the meal daily, and it will prove not only a delight, but a source of health as well as of civilisation."

By the way, dyspepsia is another name for indigestion!

What a delightful piece of advice. This voice reaches down to us through over a hundred years.

Advice about how to slow down your eating, not eat too much, and taking your time.

All these things are now coming back into practice with something that is called awareness.

On her website "Join me in the 1900's" Pat Cryer tells us this story of her mother, Florence Cole about her diet as a child around this time.

She covers the fact that, of course, there were no fridges, and food had to be cooked straight away and not kept hanging around for very long.

There was always a roast on Sunday, which is of course a tradition that has been handed down to the present day, especially in the UK. Followed on Monday by bubble and squeak (fried left over vegetables) and the leftover cold meat from Sunday. Probably the same on the Tuesday. (Although she does not mention how this was kept fresh without a fridge!)

The size of the joint was either very large or people ate smaller portions because apparently Wednesday's meal was stew and dumplings using up the rest of the Sunday joint.

The rest of the week was made up of things such as rissoles, puddings, tripe, etc.

However, we must also look at this report by Annabel Venning and Bill Mouland in the *Daily Mail* in the UK about the very poor, virtually starving children of London's East End around this time.

"They were lucky if after running around doing errands all day, they got a piece of stale bread. Older siblings would go without food to feed their younger brothers and sisters."

There is mention of Mothers' drinking gin while their children starved. There is mention of scraps of bread and cold potatoes and children being kicked to stay away from the fire where this fare was being cooked.

So we can see from this brief coverage of what food was like in the early 1900's that in a lot of cases it would only be the very well off that needed to go on a slimming diet.

The general way of eating was low in sugar and people would only have eaten small portions.

There would have been the ones who ate more, even with being poor.

I have already covered some of the tricks that were used to lose weight in the second chapter, of course.

Looking at graphs and researching brings evidence that without a doubt, obesity has risen since 1900.

As you read on you will see a gradual trend towards the problem that we have in our modern day with obesity.

A report by Huffington Post (see link below) indicates that diseases such as diabetes and heart disease have risen alongside of obesity since the 1900's. What people don't recognize is the obesity itself is not the cause of the problems, but that it is a disease that results in the bad diet that people are consuming, along with the other diseases.

We shall proceed from here into the 1910 and 1920's and see what, if any changes came about.

References.

http://www.realclearenergy.org/charticles/2012/10/01/consumer_spending_on_food_and_energy_no_longer_declining.html

http://www.1900s.org.uk/1900s-cooking.htm

http://www.huffingtonpost.ca/rachel-ryan/obesity_b_1638436.html

Chapter 4. 1910 to 1930: A Time for Some Improvement.

A report by Sandra Bradley of *Austerity Housekeeping* says that food seems to be a bit more civilised and healthy in this decade. In the typical diet of a working class family, breakfast has become an important part of the day and there is a more definite time for eating it.

There was porridge, bread-crusts in milk, (I can remember having this when I was a child in the 1940's!) bread and butter and egg, bacon, smoked haddock, hot milk and cocoa.

It is also interesting to note that this was the time that Kellogg's first invented corn flakes.

Sandra goes on to say that luncheon (a snack mid-morning) consisted of hot milk and a biscuit, or bread and butter and a banana.

Dinner (midday) consisted of soups, shepherd's pies, chops, steaks, vegetables and potatoes, steamed puddings, roly-poly (more on those in a moment) and rice or macaroni pudding, stewed fruit and custard. It's worth noting that up until about the 1960s, pasta- based and rice-based meals were unheard of.

Roly-poly was made with pastry that had been rolled out and smothered with jam, then rolled up and steamed or baked, and served with custard.

In mid-afternoon there was tea in the UK, which was bread and butter, watercress, lettuce, and stewed fruit.

At suppertime, around 7p.m., the meal consisted of bread and butter, or bread and drippings, hot milk, porridge, boiled onions, cream crackers and butter and cheese.

Moving on from Sandra's report, it is apparent that there was a lot of carbohydrate consumed in those days, but there were also a lot of vegetables and fibrous foods served, too. Meals were basically meat and vegetables, soups and stews, and bread and butter as we have already seen. The most remarkable thing is the amount that was eaten.

But it's also important to remember that people did not have centrally heated houses, and all their work was manual labour.

In the higher classes, such as landowners and the gentry or aristocracy, there were cooks and servants employed to feed the whole household.

The servants ate almost as well as the people upstairs. If you saw the TV epic Downton Abbey, you will have gotten some idea of what this was like. Remembering again of course, that the servants were often on the go from 5 a.m. until 10 p.m.

Whilst the poor were eating bread and butter, potatoes and puddings, it seems that the rich were dining on meat, fish, and a lot of cakes and sweet things. Food would have been prepared in a different way, by making eggs into soufflés for example.

The sugar intake was much lower than today as it was an expensive item, but treacle and syrup were in abundance. Probably because these were seen as the detritus that was left over from the process of refining the sugar.

Have you ever heard of Junket? This was made from sweetened milk and rennet, which is a digestive enzyme taken from the stomach of a cow. These days, apparently you can obtain a vegetarian version.

To make it, you warm the milk to a body temperature, add the rennet and leave it until it sets. Temperature is very important.

Apparently, children used to eat a lot of this, particularly children recovering from illness, as it was considered to be good for them. (Again, I can remember eating it in the forties.)

Also at this time, children were given supplements of milk, sugar, butter and watercress to help with their growth as a result of finding out the importance of minerals in the diet. Meat was also found to have first-class protein and minerals such as iron and zinc. Children from poorer families did not grow so well.

Moving on to the 1920s, things begin to change again. It is amazing how quickly things moved with the food situation in this era. Which is a good thing because, after all, we need food to survive!

According to a report about America, on 1920-30.com, food was plentiful and cheap, because of the large quantities produced by American farms. The diet was mainly meat and potatoes.

Also, because of the discovery of the importance of vitamins in 1912, fruit, vegetables and milk became much more important.

An interesting point made in this report is that eating habits changed as they ate *fewer* starches, but there was an increased consumption of fruit and sugar. This is a bit of an anomaly really, as of course, starches turn to sugar in the body anyway.

This was also the time when processed foods began making an appearance. Ready-to-cook foods became available, along with canned and frozen foods. (Although I would not put canned and frozen foods in the processed category, unless there were additives of some sort, with the exception of certain preservatives.)

According to Michelle Meadows, in her report, *A Century of Ensuring Safe Foods and Cosmetics* written in 2006, Harvey Wiley M.D. was appropriated funds by Congress to look into what was being put into foods in the way of preservatives. This was a crucial prelude to the enactment of the Food and Drugs Act of 1906, and labelling and identifying what was in foods developed throughout these two decades.

According to www.macfisheries.co.uk, the UK was also watching out for preservatives in processed foods.

Gas stoves and refrigerators were making their entrance into ordinary households. So with better transport, roads and storage, food began its journey into the modern age that we have today.

The WI ran a correspondence cooking course on how to prepare, cook and serve food using the most up-to-date information. This would have been by post, of course.

It is ironic that now in the 2010's they are doing the same thing, but online or in special classes.

Another food which was consumed a lot were rabbits. They were easy to shoot because of their large numbers, and cheap to buy for city dwellers.

The first manufactured foods included things like candy bars, "Wonder" bread, chocolate drinks, and certain cakes. There was even a big debate going on over white bread versus brown!

Other foods that we would recognise today, almost 100 years later, included Campbell's oxtail soup, Heinz tomato ketchup, Heinz spaghetti, peanut butter, instant coffee and Del Monte canned fruit and vegetables.

By 1927, adverts were seen for Campbell's vegetable and beef soup, Maxwell house coffee, Colman's mustard, bottled soda, and bouillon cubes.

My mother has lived so far to the age of 93, and keeps in good health, other than a few limitations that we would expect at her age. She has always been healthy and still lives a reasonably healthy life. She is always telling the story of how poor they were as children in this decade, but the one thing that their father always told them was that they could always help themselves to anything they liked fresh from the garden.

As it happened, he was a keen gardener, but he was doing what he could to make sure that his family never starved during their lean times. He, too, lived without illness and used to pride himself on not having to see a doctor, right up until he developed a heart complaint at the age of 81, shortly before he died. He would never eat anything that he could not check out what the ingredients were. He was lucky to have lived with a keen cook, my grandmother.

It was in 1920 that Charles Birdseye started to deep freeze food, including vegetables, fruits, fish and meats.

When prohibition came along in 1920, soft drinks also began to make a huge impact.

A company called Horn & Hardart were apparently the pioneers of the fast food industry, and they advertised on the radio that they were "Less work for mother," Which of course, made sense at the time.

In modern times, these fast foods are more for everyone's convenience though, not just mother.

When we come to look at the UK, things were not progressing as fast as in America. But they were not so far behind. Here, they ate more in the way of meat and fish than they did in the 1950's. And the amount of dairy products, cereal and fruit increased along with the amount of fat and sugar.

What is remarkable though, is that most of this was fresh to start with, but as the variety of canned and frozen foods increased, so the consumption of fresh food decreased.

New foods making an appearance were self-rising flour, baking powder, margarine and custard powder.

Breakfast was taking on a new look with cereals and the Shredded Wheat company opened a factory in London.

Instant coffee made its first appearance.

Recipes included one for sheep's head soup, rissoles, and Battenberg cake.

The financially well off still had their cooks, and far superior cuisine, such as two-tier lemon pudding, watercress salad or sandwiches, cherry tomatoes and vermicelli soufflé. The British as a whole loved their steak and kidney puddings and veal and ham pies.

Dieting to lose weight took off in strength in the 1920s. I wonder, was it coincidence that was also the time when sugar and fat were on the increase?

Although the word calorie had been around for some time, in the study of heat and energy in machines, the popularity of counting calories began in this era. Forgetting that the body is not a machine, and because scientists had been studying and measuring the heat (energy) value of foods, along with discovering vitamins and minerals and their importance. It was a Polish biochemist in 1912, working in England who proposed the vitamin theory, and by 1929 Eijkman and Hopkins received the Nobel Prize for their vitamin discoveries.

The study and development of vitamins were to progress right up to the present day.

The importance of minerals did not start to be investigated until the 1920s. Interest in calories started by measuring the energy, first for livestock and later for humans. A scientist named Atwater in the 19th century had studied the energy requirements of the body at rest. This knowledge was never proved or completed because of the lack of answers about how food was consumed.

You can read more on the links below. The point is that during the 1920s the idea of counting calories caught on.

Atwater had studied a great deal about energy consumption among manual workers and whilst his studies were never really completed, the idea caught on, and moved into the industrial market.

He left us with the idea that a woman using light exercise needed 2300 calories a day and men with the same amount of activity required 2830.

You can find many articles and advice telling you that if you deduct 500 calories a day from the usual amount that you eat, or the amount recommended above, that you will lose a pound every seven days.

Anyone counting calories to lose weight will tell you that although the first time that they use the theory, it will work, after the second or third time of putting it back on again and using the same method, they cannot actually lose weight on this amount.

The theory supposes that a pound of fat = 3500 calories. Scientifically that is correct, but this does not take into account the person who has successfully lost weight on that amount and then puts it back on again when they start eating more. Because their body cannot differentiate between the two, it has confused the cut in calories with a famine and has started preserving all the fat that it can. So for every diet that you go on, counting calories in this way, the calorie allowance goes down and down.

Imagine then what happens when you find that your calorie allowance has now gone down to 1250 a day and you cannot lose weight. Are you to cut down to 750? Think about it and you will see why being a slave to counting calories does not work.

There is a good deal of controversy going on about the subject of calories because of this. For many years, people who struggled to lose weight this way were not believed or heard, and they were accused by various bodies of eating amnesia, or telling lies, or miscounting their calories.

A Dr. H. Robert Rose wrote the following quote:

"I can't reduce my weight," is a statement scientifically absurd.

And:

"The stout person must learn that he has both friends and enemies at the table. His enemies are sugar, bread, cereal, desserts, butter, cream, olive oil, bacon, cocoa and rich sauces. Among his friends are lean meats, unsweetened fruits and green foods. Yet, alas! Most people seem stricken with an ardent love for their enemies."

References.

http://www.rd.com/slideshows/weight-loss-advice-from-1920-does-it-still-hold-up-today/

https://austerityhousekeeping.wordpress.com/2013/01/31/healthy-diets-the-1910-way/

http://www.euro.who.int/__data/assets/pdf_file/0005/96458/QU14598EU.pdf

http://www.1920-30.com/food/

http://www.fda.gov/AboutFDA/WhatWeDo/History/FOrgsHistory/CFSAN/ucm083863.htm

http://www.macfisheries.co.uk/page15.htm

http://ed-bites.blogspot.co.uk/2009/04/history-of-calorie-in-nutrition.html

http://www.chemheritage.org/discover/media/magazine/articles/29-1-counting-calories.aspx

Chapter 5. 1930's & 1940's: 2 Decades of Food Shortages and Rationing.

I have amalgamated these two decades for reasons that will become clearer as we progress.

Considering that when we look back over history we have always seen the 1930's as the time of the Great Depression, there was a surprising variety of foods. I do realise of course that it depended on where you lived, what class you were in, and also bearing in mind that people spent a higher percentage of their income on food then.

Recalling the previous discussion, material possessions had not yet taken over their priorities, whilst in our modern day, we expect to have a television, freezer, computer, etc., as an essential part of our existence. In those days, life was lived in a very simple manner.

It seems that, contrary to popular belief, during the Great Depression, there was an ample food supply.

People were willing to eat less expensive grades of meat such as chuck, rather than sirloin, beef, hearts, brains, feet etc.

People who needed help were served from soup kitchens and government programmes.

This was a decade of cutting back, but not starvation.

Magazines still published recipes and only occasionally ran an article on economical meals. Americans as well as the British did not eat out as a rule, but they did used to enjoy a coffee or a beer. I have witnessed a big change in public bars myself over the years, from a place where the men went to drink beer, to somewhere with family rooms and bar menus for eating choices. In the 30's the pub was sacred to the beer and alcohol.

Sugar prices too, were low, and bread was usually homemade. Conjure up the picture in films of people collecting a sack of flour for a month from the local outlet store!

A quote from foodtimeline.org says:

"But weren't many Americans starving in the thirties? Not really. There was hunger of course, but it was primarily concentrated in the poorest areas…And while the Dust Bowl housewives might have had to make their bread inside a drawer to keep the drifting dust out, at least there was bread. Relief agencies and make-work jobs helped some of the worst off, and low food prices made everyone except the food companies happier."

And:

"Sugar prices, too, were low, and in the thirties Americans consumed more sugar per capita than they have done before or since…" Taken *from ---Fashionable Food: Seven Decades of Food Fads, Sylvia Lovegren. Macmillan; New York. 1995 (p. 41-44)*

Note that this book is now twenty years old. I wonder if that statement still stands true today?

Foods such as baked bean sandwiches, beef stew, tongue, liver and bacon were popular, and apparently, people were still consuming in the region of 2700 calories a day.

The soup kitchens were put on by various organisations and these often offered cakes and pastries too. Probably baked by the women of the WI or the WVS. (Women's Institute and the Women's Voluntary Service.)

Both of these organisations were around in these two decades, faithfully serving tea, biscuits, soup and sandwiches to the population, in the time of food shortages and during the war. They would appear as if by magic when there was a need for sustenance to families that had been made homeless by the bombing and the workers rescuing them and putting out the fires.

The better off farmers and large land owners used to donate fruit and vegetables in season, too.

An old cookbook written by Evelyne White and Jessie R Watson called *"A Collection of Menus and Recipes for Every Day of the Year"*, which appears to be in circulation around the 1930's, has some interesting menus in it, including such items as porridge, milk, bacon, tomatoes, veal cutlets, boiled potatoes, marmalade pudding, baked beans on toast, salmon, green salad, cheese and biscuits, pigeon pie, egg patties, creamed chicken, lemon buns, stewed rhubarb and cold ham.

Another book by Ida Bailey Allen called *Cooking, Menus, Service,* in print in 1935 suggests the following menus:

Breakfast; Stewed prunes, cornflakes and milk, boiled eggs, toast and butter, coffee, milk, or oatmeal cooked with dates, top milk, bacon, muffins and butter, coffee, milk.

Lunch; Poached eggs with rice and cheese, bread and butter, grape jelly (jam to us Brits,) cocoa or Boston baked beans, steamed brown bread and butter, piccalilli, canned peaches and tea.

For a snack; Peanut butter sandwiches, or scrambled egg sandwiches, gingerbread, an apple, and cold milk or creamed chicken, ham or veal sandwiches, jelly (or jam) sandwiches and hard-boiled egg, sponge cake and lemonade.

Lunch was; Sandwiches, made with eggs or meat, followed by apple pie, cheese, coffee and an orange.

Evenings included such foods as various meats, vegetables, potatoes, fish and apple pie again.

So what about slimming diets and obesity then?

Dieting became really popular in the 1930s, but this would have only been for the better off. The working classes were hard pressed to find food, let alone worry about their weight.

Many of you will have heard about the grapefruit diet, with which it is claimed that there are enzymes in grapefruit that burn fat. But the only claim that grapefruit has to helping with weight management is that it is a fairly low calorie and lower (as opposed to low!) in sugar fruit. (Fructose) It has plenty of Vitamin C. Unfortunately, it is also quite sour and most people need it to be sweetened. So what would they sweeten it with? Sugar, of course. Thus cancelling out the good that the grapefruit would do. All the same, this became very popular.

Also, this is the decade when Ryvita was born. This was and still is a crisp-bread. In its earlier days it was simply a Rye crisp-bread. This crisp-bread was exploited as a slimming product and indeed still is to a certain extent. Though these days it is promoted more for healthy eating, and there are also numerous varieties of flavours and sizes.

It seems that the middle classes and stars (celebrities in modern jargon) were the ones who were most concerned about their shape and weight.

Stars such as Jean Harlow, Greta Garbo and Bette Davis struggled to keep their weight down by any means available. There were weight loss camps for the better off, much in the style these days of people going to a health farm.

There was a product called Bile Beans around at the time, and although these were for digestive problems, people somehow got the idea into their heads that they would be good for weight loss. They acted on the body just like a laxative.

We can see then that the need to be controlling weight with dieting was around in the 1930's, and although poorer people were not aware of the idea of keeping slim through deprivation, the financially well off and people in the limelight certainly were.

The difference between then and now is that we have more means at our disposal, and a vast variety of foods that purport to have weight reducing properties. We also have the internet and the media and a vast array of diets. I have reviewed 25 of them in my book, *How to spot the best diet. Amazon Kindle.*

My purpose in writing that book was to help people to find the best diet that will be good for them in the long run.

With the 1940s there were other big changes in people's food, weight and diet, simply because from 1939 to 1945 war broke out in most parts of the world. So the idea of dieting to lose weight was not a popular pastime, in fact, it never even entered people's minds. There was rationing and shortage of food generally, so the thought of what was fattening was far from people's minds.

Great Britain suffered the deprivation in a big way, because of the fact that they are an island, and depended on shipping to bring in supplies. The ships were under attack from enemy U-boats because of the war. What is more, because of rationing, the deprivation went on right into the 50s which by then had affected other parts of the world, too.

People were issued ration books for all sorts of items, not just food. The books contained coupons for each person in a household, and every time you bought anything that was on ration, then you had to use a coupon.

Another fact to take into account was that people were getting plenty of exercise, because they used to walk and cycle more during the war with petrol shortages.

So let's take a look at a list of foods and the amounts that people ate during the forties and up until the early 50s.

A list of the _weekly_ (not daily!) rations looked like this;

- Bacon & Ham 4 oz. (113 grams)

- Meat. ½ lb (226 grams)

- Butter 2 oz (50grams)

- Cheese 2 oz

- Margarine 4 oz

- Cooking fat (lard) 4 oz

- Milk 3 pints. (Around 1 and ½ litres)

- Sugar 8 oz

- Preserves 1 lb a month.

- Tea 2 oz

- Eggs 1 a week.

- Sweets/Candy 12oz every 4 weeks

Let me ask you to really study this list in great detail. Imagine that you can only have **one piece of cheese the size of a match box a week!** That is the size of one piece of cheese to have with your biscuits for your dessert these days!

To give you an example of how much food was rationed, my mother got married in 1943. The neighbours all collected their rations of dried fruit, sugar, butter and flour and pooled them and gave them to her mother to make the wedding cake!

White flour was in short supply and brown whole-meal flour was being used instead. Vegetables and local fruits were in a reasonable supply, because people were making an effort to grow their own.

In a PDF called *European food and nutrition policies in action. Page 19.* (Euro. who. Link below) the WHO said this:

"To everybody's astonishment, when stillbirth rates or children's weights and heights were monitored and when the disease patterns of adults were checked, it became clear that the people of Europe were often better fed during than before the Second World War." From this report I think that it is remarkable how much the government was taking an interest in people's nutritional needs.

However, things were not so rosy as they seemed. Some children born in this era were indeed suffering from malnourishment. I will discuss this in the next chapter about the 50s.

Recently, people are taking an interest in how people ate during this time, because obesity became quite a rarity. Even doctors lost interest in obesity and people were a lot smaller in stature and girth generally. There are not even any obesity statistics around for comparison. Then, in the 1950s after fourteen years of this way of eating, things began to change. There was more food around, and as a result, people were getting bigger in stature as well as girth.

It may be worth noting here that the so-called Baby Boomers generation, those born between 1948 and 1960 are the ones who have seen the biggest changes in history with diet. They have witnessed eating nothing but real food to eating the Frankenstein foods now being produced. And now in the 2010s we are seeing a vast change in health and well-being. But it is never too late to change your lifestyle, and if you are among this generation, there is still time to do something about it.

References.

http://www.foodtimeline.org/fooddecades.html

http://www.euro.who.int/__data/assets/pdf_file/0005/96458/QU14598 EU.pdf

Chapter 6. 1950s: Things Improve and Abundance Returns.

This era is the time when the phrase "Baby Boomers" was invented. The reason for this was because from round about the time of the end of the Second World War, people were getting their lives back together, men from the forces were returning home, and the economy was improving in the Western world. So at this time there was a boom in babies. At the end of the 50s the government found themselves having to cater for these babies by finding extra schools and housing.

The Baby Boomers are the ones that have seen the biggest changes in history where food and diet are concerned. And the 50s were the beginning of this change.

They are now in their sixties, an age that is showing the results in health from the deprivation of the 30s and 40s. For although there was very little obesity around, the foundations were being laid for the increase in heart disease and other illnesses that we are seeing now.

Interestingly, it was in 1948, just before this decade began, that the World Health Organisation (WHO) was formed with the idea of making food attainable to all parts of the world. The WHO had and still has a duty to make sure that food is healthy and that there is enough.

At around this time there was a study by Ancel Keys, which had found a connection with heart disease and saturated fat. Later, when we come to look at chapter 7 and the 70s, we shall see that this study was to become controversial. But at this time it was the beginning of the concern about fat causing obesity as well as heart disease.

The WHO would be keeping an eye on our food right across the board, from how it is grown or reared to the moment it hit the shopping basket of the 1950s to the supermarket trolleys of today.

But the WHO was still in its infancy and stated that much further research was needed, before public health authorities could recommend major alterations in the diet or were justified in advising that more or less of any particular kind of fat would be beneficial.

So it seems that although it had been brought to the WHO's attention, they felt that they could not recommend anything until it was scientifically proven. Therefore, it is not an easy task for any of us to know who we can trust where eating is concerned. Because it can take many decades for science to prove anything where health comes into question and research, authorities can be just standing around waiting and watching as nations sink into unhealthy eating and habits.

For example, when I first started researching and studying diet and weight in the 1980s there was a book that I read at the time, and was popular in circles of people who were doing the same as me, called *"Pure White and Deadly"* written by a British professor called John Yudkin.

The book was about sugar, and the title speaks for itself. This book was ignored by the experts and authorities at the time and put down to a type of quackery, but this is what Robert Lustig has to say in an article written for the Telegraph on the day that I am writing this. (Link below)

"Without even knowing it, I was a Yudkin acolyte. Everything this man said in 1972 was the God's honest truth and if you want to read a true prophecy you find this book... I'm telling you every single thing this guy said has come to pass. I'm in awe."

This information took forty years to be recognised because of the lack of proof.

I do understand of course that authorities cannot just go along with every idea, but I do wonder why when people who study the subject carefully and put a lot of work into their own research, like Professor Yudkin, are just ignored.

This is what is happening at the moment with the current controversy over saturated fat causing heart disease. But we will discuss that more as we work our way through the next few decades.

Foods that we take for granted now in 2015, were not around then in the UK in the 1950s.

Among them are curry, pasta, many spices and herbs, pizza and Chinese food. The word "takeaway" was unheard of and the only ready-made food you bought in the shops was fish and chips, which were wrapped in newspaper lined with grease-proof bag to stop the ink from getting into the food, or pies and pasties. Ready-made cakes were now becoming more popular.

Rice was a milk pudding; bread and butter were an everyday food. My brother used to love rice pudding, which was made by putting about 2 oz of rice into 1 pint of milk, two tablespoons of sugar and a knob of butter. Place in the oven and cook for 90 minutes in a moderately hot oven. So it tended to be put into the oven at the same time as the meat for the Sunday roast.

He loved it so much, that my mother challenged him one day and said that she would make one for him all to himself, and dared him to eat it all. He did!

Vegetables were carrots, turnips, parsnips, and sprouts or kale and potatoes. Olive oil was kept in the medicine cabinet, and you used lard or dripping for frying. Eating raw fish would not have been considered healthy. Sushi would only have been known in Japan.

Figs and dates were something that you ate at Christmas. Ice cream came in either vanilla or as a luxury there would be strawberry flavour. Jelly and ice cream were party foods. Crisps were one flavour with a small blue packet of salt in the bag and were something you bought yourself with pocket money. There was one type of cheese, and that was a cheddar.

Hot cross buns were eaten only on Good Friday, and you had one hollow Easter egg, on Easter Sunday morning. Milk was not pasteurised and families fought over who was going to have the cream from the top of the bottle. My mother used to scald the cream to make clotted cream.

Food was purchased from the local shops, supermarkets were unheard of. I remember shopping with my mother, going from one type of shop to another because food was not all under the same roof.

We went to the Baker for bread, Grocer for cheese and eggs, (I can still smell it!) and the Green Grocer for fruit and vegetables. The Butcher was where you bought the meat. Shopping was a daily occurrence as we did not have a refrigerator. Milk was delivered by a milkman, which was a tradition carried on for many years and still is in some rural parts of the UK.

Sainsbury's was the first to try out a supermarket in the UK in 1957.

Another noticeable thing was that fruit and vegetables and some other foods, were seasonal. You would have been very surprised to find a lettuce in the middle of winter, or a turnip in the middle of summer. Strawberries were only available in May, June and July.

Apples tasted delicious. The Granny Smiths in September every year were something to look forward to, as were the Cox's apples and the russets. Crisp, fresh and tasty.

There would have been no such thing as grazing in front of the television, simply because television was rare in those days. Snacks were something that you took to work or school for midmorning.

Breakfast would have been porridge or cornflakes or toast and marmalade and sometimes an egg.

Lunch might have been sandwiches filled with meat-paste or corned beef, or egg. Soup was popular for lunch times, too. Salad would have consisted of lettuce, tomato, cucumber and maybe a little watercress. This was the time when salad cream came into its own.

However, many working class people had the main meal of the day at lunch time (known as dinner) and such meals as cottage pie, pasties, pies, steak and kidney pudding, sausage and mash and on Sunday, the proverbial roast. Chicken was a luxury and many people had this for their Christmas dinner. Turkey was a rarity.

Mary, who was a child in that decade, told me of the chicken that her family had as a pet, and they had the benefit of her eggs for eating. This chicken, who the family fondly called Cynthia, used to sit on her aunt's head while she did the ironing, to the amusement of the kids in the family. One day, Cynthia was missing and they never saw her again, no explanation and no sign of her anywhere. Was it coincidence that a couple of days later, there was chicken for dinner? They never found out, it was the aunt's secret.

No home was complete without the jam, syrup, tomato sauce, brown sauce and mustard in the cupboard. There would be no other condiments, except if there was some pickle, piccalilli or home-made pickled onions.

Something that emerged in the early years of this decade was that many children were still suffering from the ravages of shortage during the rationing.

Chris, now aged 66, said that as a child, he had to wear leg braces, (we used to call them leg irons) for many years after suffering from rickets. Which is a shortage of vitamin D and calcium. When he went into the Marines, many years later they put him down as malnourished.

Now in his 60s he is suffering a form of leukemia, atrial fibrillation and rheumatoid arthritis.

It may be worth noting here, that in 2015 we are seeing a return of this problem in children as they are not getting enough Vitamin D or calcium. Both of these nutrients are obtained from oily fish and sunlight. The modern diet and the fear that has been instilled in people of sunlight has brought about the return of this awful disease.

The difference between now and the 50s diet is that although we have plenty of food around in the western world, we are eating the wrong kinds of food. With empty calories and no nourishment in the Frankenstein foods that are being produced.

Chris's story is why we need to be more careful of watching our children's diet. They can become malnourished just as much through eating a diet of chicken nuggets and chips, crisps and candies as through not eating anything.

Women burned up a lot more calories in their everyday lives in the 50s. Washing machines were not in general use, and all the washing was done by boiling the whites in the "copper" and lifting them out with wooden tongs and, dropping them into the sink. Then pummelling them and putting them through a wringer. No tumble dryer, but there would be the physical action of hanging them out on the line to dry. So washing the clothes was a workout in itself, besides all the other chores to be got through in a day.

When she got married, a friend of mine had a concerned phone call from her mother on washing day to find out how she got on hanging out the clothes on the line, and particularly concerned about how she managed the sheets! Imagine the energy you burnt lifting heavy wet sheets up over a line and pulling the line up to a suitable height.

Homes were not centrally heated and calories were used up just to keep warm.

You walked or cycled everywhere, including the shopping expedition. Children walked to and from school, then went out to play, skipping, chasing and playing ball games.

The midmorning break would have been coffee (Camp which was made out of barley and coffee flavouring in the UK) with a biscuit. Not a heavy calorie-laden snack that we would have today.

Things looked a little different on the other side of the Atlantic at that time though.

In a list from an article called *"What were Americans cooking in the 1950s?"* appetizers are mentioned. This was unheard of in the UK except among the better off. People would not have needed their appetite to be stimulated, they were hungry enough!

Among them, I found such items as fruit cup, Melon ball cocktail, Sea food cocktail, Pastry snails, silver dollar hamburgers, bacon wraparounds. Followed by about 30 more choices.

Another 30 or more different soups and salads, including for the soups, tomato, chicken and corn, onion, oxtail, cream of celery. And for the salads, stuffed tomato, three- bean, orange and Bermuda onion, coleslaw and cold potato salad.

Main courses consisted of grilled kabobs, scalloped chicken supreme, beef and corn casserole, American lasagne, fluffy meat loaf and baked ham with glaze. Salmon steak, chicken a-la-king, spaghetti with sauce and ham and vegetable casserole.

Vegetables were often served with butter, cream sauce, sour cream sauce, canned soup, and topped with breadcrumbs or dried onion flakes.

Desserts consisted of such items as chiffon pie, coconut cake, peppermint candy, cake, banana chiffon cake, apricot soufflé and banana chocolate cake.

Those were the days of the first barbecues in America, too. While the Brits were still tucking into their fish and chips from wrapped in newspaper while walking along Blackpool front, or baking potatoes at the camp fire, the Americans were setting up their barbecues and cooking the steaks and chicken wings, and barbecued ribs. Certainly worlds apart from the UK.

On the subject of fish and chips, children were often given a penny to go to the fish and chip shop for a bag of "scraps". These were the bits that came off the fish while being cooked in the deep fat fryers, and came to the surface when they were being cleaned!

The 1950s brought about more changes in the way that we saw cooking. It became a chore and something that just had to be done in the quickest and shortest way possible. (A habit that I still have, but at least I do it with real food!)

In the 50s dieting was seen as something to make you more attractive and to obtain a lovely figure. Women were happier to be a bigger size than in the later years. An icon of the fifties, Marilyn Monroe was a size 14 (or American size 12.) She was known for her hourglass figure and for her beauty.

This was an era when lower fat foods started appearing on the market, but the emphasis was on naturally lower fat foods and not foods that were specially made.

The word "fitness" was not used for many years yet, and exercise was something you did as a pastime. Exercises were known as procedures rather than routines.

I well remember a dieting product called AYDS which involved eating a sort of toffee before you had your meal, which was supposed to fill you up and take away your appetite!

Did it work? What do you think?

But I was daft enough to try it when I came to dieting in the 1960s. The makers claimed that you could lose a pound a day! In those days, advertising was not so strictly monitored, but this is an example of why it became necessary to monitor it more closely.

Another example of a typical way of dieting was a book being sold and delivered to people, under plain wrapper. It was called *The New Way to Eat and Get Slim.* by Donald G. Cooley. He claimed that by following this *scientific* method, you could lose weight without:

1. Denying yourself

2. The drudgery of exercise

3. Drugs, pills or compounds

4. Steam baths or massage.

From this, we can see how losing weight was considered quite a battle, and this book was promising women their freedom from all this. (Link below under hathitrust.)

It has many good points in it such as the quality and type of calories, but it is based very much on calorie intake. It looks very familiar to me, as it is exactly what I used to do with diets in the early 60s. What he does not take into account, and of course would not have realised, was that when you finish the diet, your metabolism is lower. He actually says *that when the desired weight is lost, then you must stop the diet.*

At this time, there was a lot of emphasis placed on being slim for your husband. This brings to mind the memory that it was widely accepted that you got fatter after getting married and having children. The expectation then was that you were seen as beautiful and attractive in order to win a husband. Once you were married, it was part of the journey of life that you accepted shortage of money and nice clothes along with losing your figure, as part of being a married woman.

Women used props for helping them to keep their tummy in; it was the known practice that before you had children you wore a little suspender belt to keep your stockings up, but afterwards you progressed to a corset!

Amphetamines were a way of keeping weight down too. In fact, some doctors started to prescribe them as part of their private practice. Although often, the prescription would be for other health matters, but became known as "Mother's little helper."

Cigarettes became a prop for keeping weight down too and were actually used as part of some cigarette advertising. To this day, many people are afraid of giving up smoking for that reason. But it is a myth that you replace the food with a cigarette. People usually end up with both!

Everyday portion sizes were smaller then and so were the women. An average waist size in the 50s was 27 inches. Nowadays it is 32. But the irony is that it was considered to be just as bad to be too thin as it was to be too fat. Women used to wear padding inside their clothing to make them look bigger and you would be teased if your friends found out you were wearing a padded bra.

The average height for women in the 50s was 5ft.2in and she wore a size 12 dress. (Jeans had not yet come into vogue, and trousers were not worn as a matter of course.) She measured 37 bust 27 waist and 39 hips. There was much emphasis on these measurements.

If you were "off" your food in those days, you went to the doctors to have a tonic prescribed, "To increase your appetite!"

One popular film star around at this time was Diana Dors. Her famous dimensions were 35-25-35. But unfortunately, keeping to her trim figure was costly, because as she got older she put on a lot of weight after battling with marital difficulties and cancer.

She went on to become a diet celebrity on British Television and made a video and had her own diet book. Sadly, the battle with cancer had to take first place and she lost the battle altogether when she died at the age of 52.

At the end of the 50s and into the 60s things really began to change on the food and diet front.

References:

Arterial hypertension and ischemic heart disease: preventive aspects. Report of an Expert Committee. Geneva, World Health Organization, 1962 (WHO Technical Report Series, No. 231).

http://www.foodtimeline.org/fooddecades.html

http://babel.hathitrust.org/cgi/pt?id=coo.31924090162201;view=1up;seq=75

Chapter 7. 1960's: A New Freedom.

As we work our way through the 20th century, it is becoming more and more clear that self-image and beauty did not include accepting being fat or overweight. The word obese was never used by the public, only in medical circles. You were simply too fat.

By the 1960s unemployment was very low and the western world had at long last recovered from the rationing of the Second World War. Along with this came a big change in the way that people ate. Television was more popular with people able to afford to buy them and with it came the cooks and their cookery programmes.

Fanny Craddock was the TV cook of the day, and she had her husband running around behind her in the studio, much to the viewer's amusement.

People started taking more holidays abroad and in turn, there were more visitors coming to the UK. The British particularly were being influenced by ideas from abroad. Italian dishes, such as spaghetti Bolognese were taken on as part of everyday eating.

Chinese takeaways began to spring up in competition with the fish and chip shops. Indian restaurants began to make an appearance. But in spite of that, fish and chips remained a British favourite for a long time to come.

Meat and sugar consumption reached an unprecedented level. Tinned or canned foods became more popular.

One of the biggest revolutions was the large, white, sliced loaf of bread. There was intense competition between firms for the best white bread. A soft, doughy consistency, but nevertheless very popular because of its convenience.

Cereals started to take on a whole new look with sugar being added to them. Where before people were content with puffed wheat, now it was reinvented as sugar puffs.

A much greater variety of foods were available, and supermarkets had taken off, getting bigger and bigger. Sainsbury's doubled its number of food products from 2000 to 4000 over the decade.

Air travel meant that we could import more foods, including fruit and vegetables. By the end of the decade, the wonderful seasonal Granny Smith apple became an all year round fruit and never tasted the same again. We could get tomatoes in the winter and the avocado made an appearance.

Frozen food shops and stores started to appear and frozen foods became everyday items. Part of a family's budget was now spent on a freezer in the home.

Not only did supermarkets change the way we shopped, but they began to change what we ate. The 60s heralded in the new way of packaging and longer life on the shelves, thereby making more preservatives necessary.

Recipes that defined the 60s were such foods as tinned peaches in a jelly mold, prawn cocktail, meatballs, chicken a-la-king, fondue, beef Bourguignon. Prawn cocktail was a popular starter when eating out.

It was at this time that new types of health problems started to emerge; heart disease and cancer of the breast, lung and large bowel. Was this the result of eating more refined foods which had been introduced at first as luxury foods, but soon became a way of eating that was normal? Bearing in mind the fluffy white loaf!

During the Second World War, people were concentrating and being educated on what was nutritious, but now the government was losing its control over our food choices. The food industry had become a vast influence because they were being included as members on the panels of controlling bodies such as the WHO and the FDA (Food and Drug Administration.)

The 60s also brought about a change in fashion. Miniskirts, a dress called the sack, which is a good description, tights or pantyhose were introduced, denim jeans became popular, 3-inch heels known as "stiletto" heels, and tight skirts all were in fashion.

It is quite amusing now to notice in the popular movies of that era, such as the James Bond stories, women chasing villains in their skirts and high heels. You can see them removing the shoes during the chase!

It became the trend to be stick thin and flat chested. The decade began with waists and flared skirts, but as it wore on, fashion changed and you no longer yearned for a waist less than 26 inches, but legs that were straight up and down and a dead flat stomach.

This was the time of my life when I became pregnant at the early age of 19. I really struggled with my weight at this time, and after the second pregnancy, I was the heaviest weight of the whole of my life at 14 stone.

But I pretty soon lost it, as I hated being that big. Not very big by some of today's standards, but too big for me to be happy. I lost it with an orange and peanut diet, which was popularised with Judith Chalmers, on tour around Britain giving away the diet, and free oranges and peanuts. Sponsored and brought about by Outspan Oranges.

The idea was that you ate an orange and 2 oz of peanuts for one meal a day! But it worked for me, by getting me to start watching my intake of calories. This was my first encounter with counting calories, which just ended up with lowering my metabolism. So much so that for the next forty years, and even today, I can eat only a very limited amount of food because my body still thinks it needs to preserve the calories for famine.

The irony of it is that apparently people are less interested in losing weight now than they were in the 60s. Is this because we are accepting being a larger size now? We shall look at this in a later chapter.

A survey carried out by the Department of Health said that when questioned in 1967, 9 out of 10 people attempted to lose weight, compared to just over 5 out of 10 in 2010.

This is interesting as this is not what we are led to believe. In these days of what is commonly known as "The Obesity Epidemic" we are led to believe that most people are on a diet or watching their weight.

I believe that what is actually happening is that we are more "aware" of the need to watch our weight, but not enough people are prepared to sacrifice taste and convenience for it.

In the same article above, in the 60s, only 7% of those who considered themselves to be overweight, had failed to do anything about it, compared to 43% of today's adults.

This bears out what I said earlier about there not being the pressure to lose that extra stone that people carried around. There was no BMI table to match up to.

The reason for this anomaly is that people in the 60s were not pressed to be thin in order to be acceptable as we are today. Because it is dieting in overweight people that gets them hooked into the dieting trap; they lose the ability to lose weight because of a lowered metabolism.

People were more active then because there were not so many cars, children walked to school, they played outside. Adults walked or cycled to work or the station if they were commuting.

The one main event in the world of dieting in this decade was the birth of Weight Watchers. This was started in the house of Jean Nidetch, who was fed up with being fat. There was no one to turn to and share her problems with, so she called a group of her friends over and before she knew it there were over 40 people crowding into her house.

They soon realised that losing weight would be easier if the problem was shared. This was the start of a vast empire, which eventually got taken over by the food companies, and was never the same. Unfortunately, the food company started producing foods and products to go with the classes. Many of these foods had many ingredients, in some, too many to count. The non-food products became an industry all of its own.

So the benefits of WW were watered down and soon people were simply coming along for the weigh in and not stopping for the benefits of the classes.

There were a few faddy diets around at this time, including the Knudsen 225 and the Metrecal liquid diets. These are still around in a different form, but some of them are only sold through a representative.

Then there was the Stillman Diet. This was an early version of the Atkins and Zone diet and discouraged intake of carbohydrates. But it also told people not to eat any fat and only lean protein.

This way of eating (low-fat and high protein) can lead on to problems such as cancer, high cholesterol, kidney failure, kidney stones and osteoporosis, according to Web m.d.

So we can see that the 60s was a time when dieting started to become a way that could lead to disaster for those people who were worried about weight. But there was still not the obsession with diet and exercise or the need to be stick thin, even though it was fashionable. Being thin was something that "Other people" aspired to and did not really apply to everyone.

Nevertheless, dieting became a way of life for many, including myself and we lived our lives always looking for the next new magical idea or for someone to come up with the answer.

Then along came the 70s and things began to take on an even more frightening aspect, as medical people started to tell us that we were in danger of certain illnesses if we did not lose weight!

Reference.

http://news.bbc.co.uk/1/hi/health/8538496.stm

Chapter 8. The 1970s: The Decade of the New Dietary Goals.

One of the fun things about food became very popular in the 1970s. Fondue. This consisted of a pot in the middle of the table, heated up over a flame. The pot contained either oil or some other sort of heated dip. You could also have melted chocolate for guests to dip their fruit into, which is still a popular idea these days.

The guests all had a fork each, and there were cubes of meat. You dipped the fork into the meat cubes, and dipped them into the boiling oil, to cook the cube of meat to your liking. There were variations of this with melted cheese or sauces.

The beauty of it was that it took a long time and you would while away the time chatting while you were waiting for your food to cook. It was a lot of fun and interestingly, you did not eat very much because of it.

This is because the brain apparently takes about twenty minutes to register that you are full, so that while you were busy chatting, the brain and the stomach were doing their own thing, then suddenly you realised that you could not eat any more.

Other types of food that became popular in the 70s were pasta, rice dishes, Chinese, Indian and other eastern foods. Spicy food became popular, and with that came the need for more spices in the larder.

French dressings, Waldorf salad, BBQ sauces, sweet and sour sauces, thousand-island dressing, vinaigrette, and a variety of new sauces. Sachets and tins of dressings were introduced.

So you can see that the supermarket shelves were getting bigger with the need to hold all this.

Whereas beforehand we were content with "egg and bacon pie" this became known as Quiche and different varieties and flavours were introduced.

Crisps (or chips in the USA) were transformed from the little packet with the blue bag of salt to flavours such as cheese and onion, sour cream, BBQ, chicken and so on.

Curry became very popular, and this was served with rice or fries, and sachets were sold in the supermarkets for the household cook to add to meats.

Ice cream started to have different flavours too. While people were used to either vanilla or strawberry, suddenly there was coffee, mint, rum and coke and even egg and bacon!

So far we have seen that the 70's brought about an explosion of taste. Along with this came many different additives, chemicals, artificial flavourings and a huge increase in the consumption of sugar and salt.

Another revolution was the home cocktail bar. People were drinking at home more and wine was becoming something to add to the weekly shop. It became fashionable to keep spirits and a variety of drinks in the house, and at Christmas, instead of the men disappearing to the pub on Christmas morning, they were sitting at home drinking from their own mini bars.

As the decade progressed, there were such foods as Granola, egg Mcmuffins, cups of dried noodles, (which you simply added water to) chocolate chip cookies, muller-lite yoghurts, stuffed pasta shells, different types of coffees, Perrier Water and Ben and Jerry's homemade ice cream in the popular circuit.

Dieting for weight loss had not really altered very much from the 1960s, until something of a revolution happened in 1977.

"Healthy Eating" was not really a popular concept up until this decade. Then, a certain George McGovern, former Democratic Senator, was the driving force behind the *1977 Dietary Goals for the United States. This was also known as the McGovern Report.*

At that time, animal fat intake in the USA from red meat, poultry and dairy foods was very high compared to previous intake, and coincidentally, so was heart disease and stroke, resulting in premature death.

In the book, *Functional Foods Revolution.*, Heasman and Mellentin say that at the time this report caused controversy among professionals, but by the end of the year 1977, a second and revised edition was published. (Page 62)

These authors quote a foreword from the statement as follows:

"The value of dietary change remains controversial, and science cannot at this time insure that an altered diet will provide improved protection from certain killer diseases such as heart disease and cancer."

Horseman and Mellentin went on to say that apparently among the criticisms at the time were that more research was needed, relationships were not provided, it was politically motivated, it promised the public too much, it was based too much on intuition and it was puritanical. (Page 64) Truswell, 1987.

Still in 2015, this report and everything that went with it and that has come out of it, still remains controversial. There are many studies, much research and authors and journalists, who can point the way to the fact that this report was questionable. Yet the diet since then, worldwide, has been influenced and people now believe that this way of healthy eating is Biblical!

If anyone suggests any other way, they are immediately accused of being faddy and controversial. Medical authorities will not listen to any other argument. Patients are told that this is THE way to go and that it would be more than their jobs' worth for a professional to advise you in any other way.

The McGovern report concluded that these foods; meat, saturated fat, sugars and salt, were causing these deaths as well as other diseases such as cancer, diabetes and obesity and that we should be eating more fruit, vegetables, unsaturated fat, and cereal and starchy foods.

This had the effect that people and their governments began to see food as a public health issue, with the result that the food industry developed foods that would fit in with this idea, and our shelves were filling up with low-fat foods, and numerous starchy ones.

I can remember seeing biscuits appear on the shelves that were claiming to be healthy because they were low fat. What people, including myself for a while, were failing to realise was that to make up for the lack of taste from fat, there was a big increase in the amount of sugar used.

Do you think that it could be a coincidence that since then the obesity and diabetic diseases have increased in vast numbers?

People also failed to realise that when starches are consumed, the body treats them exactly like sugar, and will store fat in exactly the same way.

But eating starchy foods is the same as eating sugar. Here is a very brief description of why.

When we eat sugar and starchy foods, to cut a very long story of the digestive process short, sugar ends up in the bloodstream. We have an organ called the pancreas, and one of its jobs is to produce insulin. This hormone processes the sugar to get it out of the bloodstream and into our fat storage cells.

Imagine a row of lockers, (the cells) and someone (the insulin) storing stuff in them until it's needed. So it is with insulin and sugar. In other words, it is storing up the sugar for energy which may come in handy at a later date. Could be hours, could be weeks or months.

The problem is that it may never be needed because of the person's inactivity or simply that they have taken on more energy than they need for their lifestyle. So guess what happens? It stays in the fat cells and keeps mounting up. Overweight and Obesity and also Type 2 Diabetes can be the result.

Robert Lustig in his book *Fat Chance* will give you a fully comprehensive explanation of this procedure.

So this dietary report was the beginning of a revolution in the 1970s that led on to the food industry taking on a huge reason to make profits and "Jump on the proverbial bandwagon."

This brought us into the next decade of the 1980s and the beginning of an obesity crisis. There are now growing numbers of people with Type 2 Diabetes that are still being told to base their meals on starchy foods!

Chapter 9. 1980s: The Food Industry Cashes In.

Some foods that made their appearance in the 1980s were Doritos, Aspartame (artificial sweetener) Lean Cuisine, (diet ready meals) and Capri-sun, (a sugary fruit drink in a pouch with a straw attached.) Also, Redbull, skittles, bagels, chicken Mcnuggets, and vegetarian burgers.

Cereals were making a big hit with different types and flavours including crunchy nut cornflakes.

This was the era of the ready meal. More and more families had two working parents, which was ironic, because while there was more money coming into the household, there was more going out on convenience foods.

The main criteria with food became that the faster you could prepare and eat it, the better. No longer was food something to be lingered over, unless you were having people to an evening meal. Even then it became the vogue to order in a Chinese takeaway or pizza delivery.

Eating out became normal for families and fast food restaurants filled up with children eating chips with everything and even then, not from plates but from paper throw away containers.

The first Pizza hut opened in the 80s and this Italian meal has become the norm and remains popular with today's lifestyle. It is quick and easy and you can eat it hot or cold. Far from recognisable as the original pizza from Italy.

Sandwiches became a hit with firms cashing in on pre-packed and prepared. Offices were surrounded by vans selling them and there were people making and delivering them.

It was the ideal way of eating that had been handed down by previous generations, from the humble meat paste or corned beef from the 40s and 50s to ever more substantial fillings like meat and salad and the favourite BLT. (Bacon, lettuce and tomato)

Life was speeding up all around, and a woman could shop in her lunch hour for clothes, household goods and food, all under one roof.

The 80s, like the 60s were a boom time and food and drink were bountiful.

Ironically, it was in this decade that the low-fat boom took off. Pasta and starchy foods became the in thing to eat. As well as being quick to prepare, it was reckoned to be healthy.

Supermarkets became out of town superstores and Sainsbury's product range grew from 7000 in 1980 to 17000 by the end of the decade.

Supermarkets became very powerful during this decade, and were certainly a big influence in the way that people ate. In the UK, where the milkman had always delivered milk every morning to people's houses by leaving their order on the doorstep, now you picked up a 4 litre container from the supermarket and kept it in the fridge or freezer.

This was the era too when skimmed and semi-skimmed milk became more popular than whole milk. Slimming clubs used to tell us that skimmed milk was better as we could drink more for our calorie allowance.

Another reason for this was because fat had become the arch enemy, thanks to the McGovern bill in the USA.

The catalyst of this was from a study and report from a man called Ancel Keys, which had led on to the McGovern report mentioned in the previous chapter. There is still some controversy about the Key's study and findings, and there is an interesting link at the end of this chapter, for you to read to see what you think for yourself.

Paleo and other researchers and writers have pointed out the flaws that were in this study, but the blame should not lie in the hands of Keys, but of the people who jumped on this bandwagon and brought about the anti-fat scare, which resulted in a billion-dollar industry in low-fat foods.

Whether Keys was right or wrong, there is still the fact that the low-fat industry did not do us any favours.

A very recent report (published the day before I wrote this) shows that saturated fat is not the demon, but high carbohydrate is.

http://www.medicalnewstoday.com/articles/285915.php

This article shows that although it could be argued that Keys got it right or wrong, it still seems that with the increased intake in carbohydrate and sugar, and the demonising of fat, we have ended up with obesity, type 2 diabetes and heart disease.

David Kessler covers this in his excellent book *"The End of Overeating"*

To this day, authorities still perpetuate this idea, with the "Eat Well" plate displayed on doctors and hospital waiting rooms.

People started and still do believe that eating low-fat foods is the norm.

Yet from this era we have inherited a standard of eating that is coinciding with a huge increase in diseases such as obesity, type 2 diabetes and heart disease.

Another development was one of back to the pills again. Drug companies were still trying to find an answer. They thought that they had found it with Phenfluramines. But unfortunately there was a connection with a fatal lung disease and people died. It had been labelled Fen-Phen and pushed as a wonder drug.

A scandal broke out over it when a Dr. Rich had made the connection. He was interviewed on a news programme in the USA about it. He very soon received a telephone call from a drug company saying that "Some very bad things would happen to him" if he said any more.

He did not pursue the matter and the pharmaceutical company denied they had ever said anything. Then the company had to defend its position when people began to sue them. By 2006 they had to set aside

21 billion dollars to compensate people, but they never did admit liability. You can find some of this story here: http://www.lawyersandsettlements.com/articles/pph_class_action/pph-lawsuits-00575.html#.VI3GKSusUV0

And here; http://www.pbs.org/wgbh/pages/frontline/shows/prescription/hazard/fenphen.html

A very popular diet of this era was also the Cambridge Diet. This provided something in the region of 500 calories a day in the form of milkshakes and liquids. These liquid diets have been around in many shapes and forms over the decades, and they are popular because of their quick fix approach.

But I want to repeat that they are not the answer, because as soon as you eat real food, the weight will come back on sooner or later. Your health will suffer very quickly if you try to live on them.

The other huge revolution in the 1980s was the fitness industry and the huge interest in exercise.

Jacques Perreti, a journalist who did a programme on British Television (BBC2 in 2012) reported that up until the diet revolution of the 1980s gyms were used by men to develop their muscles and to keep fit. They were also used by people who wanted to keep their cardiovascular systems healthy. Then the gyms saw a way to make money by advertising that people could lose weight by exercising more. Going to the gym has become a way of life now for many people.

Jacques started his programme off with this explanation about them which he was told by a gym instructor that one hour of extreme training will only burn off the equivalent of two Mars bars. That would be five hours of intense exercise a week. So in order for exercise and gyms to work for you, you also need to be eating a fairly restrictive diet.

People have run away with the idea that they can eat what they like and by going to the gym, can then burn it off. If you are a gym fan, then you may have experienced the hunger afterwards and found yourself thinking along the lines that it does not matter because I have worked hard.

Professor Wilkin of Plymouth University told Jacques, that with his research into children and exercise he found that the children were actually compensating after they had exercised and resting more. The body was making up the energy loss. It may not happen straight away; you may not be hungry for some time, but it does happen usually within a couple of days.

In his book *Instinctive Fitness,* Oliver Selway says the same. Exercise is not a good way to expect weight loss.

But in the 1980s the fitness boom was well under way. Jane Fonda, a well-known icon of the 60s made a video called *"Fitness"* and the age of Lycra and leotards was well under way. She was chosen because she had written a fitness book.

This was also the decade of health magazines and diet books gaining shelf space everywhere. Even Princess Diana was filmed going to a gym. But the photos of her were being used by the media and the gym in question was sued and went bankrupt.

In America a chap called Richard Simmons started a big business of exercise for losing weight. He did exercise classes and gave people a diet. However, his secret was not the exercise or diet, but teaching people their self-worth. He is still in business today and people love him for his character and charisma and the fact that they gained self-esteem and learnt to love themselves in order to get it right.

Now that I can absolutely go along with. Loving and valuing yourself is what it is all about.

The 90s came along then with still more changes, but more awareness of Healthy Eating.

Reference.

http://rawfoodsos.com/2011/12/22/the-truth-about-ancel-keys-weve-all-got-it-wrong/

Chapter 10. 1990s: A New Awareness Creeps In

One big thing becomes apparent when studying food and diet in the 1990s, and that is that people started to become more aware of how their eating was affecting their health.

Not only were there more diseases cropping up such as Type 2 diabetes and heart disease, but there was also an increase in digestive problems.

IBS (Irritable bowel syndrome,) allergies, food intolerances, and cancer of the colon was on the increase.

Medical authorities were in denial (and still are) but other health practitioners and nutritionists were getting alarmed and did their own studies of the problem.

People claiming that they knew the answers were coming out of the proverbial woodwork. Paleo, raw food, vegetarians, low-carbohydrate, all took their places in the frontline and prepared for battle.

The food industry was still arguing that what they were producing was okay, (just like the tobacco industry had before them) and saying that there were no good or bad foods.

In the mid-nineties a big change in perspective came about when Professor Phillip James of the Obesity Task Force advised the American government, that they needed to change the BMI safety level from 18 to 27 to 18 to 25. (Remember our discussion in chapter 3 about the BMI?)

When they did this, according to Jacques Perretti, it immediately made 29 million people overweight overnight! The ripple effect of this was world-wide. Which in turn turned these people into consumers for the diet industry.

Slimming clubs, gyms, food consortiums all cashed in on the act and the diet industry was huge. They went from a 30-billion dollar industry to double that amount in ten years.

Such items as Kellogg's Special K, became big bucks. It went from being just a breakfast cereal to a diet in itself. Women were targeted with adverts such as the bikini, and the little red dress. Can you pinch an inch? Well, yes I bet anyone but the skinniest can pinch an inch just above their waists. But this became a reason to diet. Yet Special K alone became a 1.7 billion dollar industry.

As Jacques said, all this was aspirational but was it attainable? According to my memory, it certainly was not. It developed into an era of neurotic dieting and brought about a serious epidemic of eating disorders and eventually an overweight and obesity nightmare.

People's lives were being made a misery over a mere seven pounds in weight!

As the decade wore on and people started to become interested in healthy eating, this brought about the advent of the Health Food Shop. At first, they were the only places where you were presented with shelves of foods claiming to be free from the products that seemed to be doing harm, such as gluten free breads, (the first ones produced were horrible and the only way that you could eat the bread was by toasting it!) gluten free biscuits, dairy free yoghurts, etc.

Meanwhile, the shelves in the supermarket were getting bigger and bigger, laden down with sugary foods. They also started to realise the demand for alternative gluten-free and dairy-free foods, but many of them contained sugar and fat.

Nuts were becoming a problem for many kids. Suddenly the labelling said that foods either did or did not contain nuts, particularly peanuts.

It may be worth noting at this point that there is a big difference between allergies with certain foods, and being intolerant to them.

An allergy will bring on an anaphylactic attack, which can be fatal if not treated urgently. Whereas a food intolerance simply causes bloating or digestive problems or other discomfort.

In the 1980s I remember visiting the Epcot Centre in Disneyland, Florida and seeing a projected layout of what farming in the future would look like. There were vast, open prairies of wheat and grains being grown and someone in a control box, controlling the machinery as it harvested the crops. While we have not exactly come to that, during the 90s we certainly headed towards it at a rapid rate.

Farmers were being controlled by vast food consortiums and being told what and how they could grow their crops and how to look after livestock.

Foods from all over the world, and consequently often out of season were appearing. Tropical fruits were available in cold climates, root vegetables during hot weather. Often, fruits were delivered to the supermarket and not ripe. It became normal for people to buy fruit to ripen at home, but many times as soon as the fruit ripened, it rotted away within a couple of days.

The farmers growing and producing foods were going out of pocket. As supermarkets made vast profits while paying the source only a small fraction of the cost to the consumer.

It is reckoned that the average consumption of calories in the 90s had doubled since the 70s

The nineties also saw an inconsistency in the way that Governments were advising people.

This is a list taken from *The Functional Foods Revolution* that they took from a guide published in the UK by the Health Education Authority entitled *The Balance of Good Health.* Page 66.

1. *Enjoy your food;*

2. *Eat a variety of different foods;*

3. *Eat the right amount to be a healthy weight;*

4. *Eat plenty of foods rich in starch and fibre;*

5. *Eat plenty of fruit and vegetables;*

6. *Don't eat too many foods that contain a lot of fat;*

7. *Don't eat sugary foods and drinks too often;*

8. *If you drink alcohol, drink sensibly;*

This guide smacks of a cop out! It does not really give anyone who is not familiar with good wholesome food a guide for how to eat in a healthy way. The reason for that is all about how politics played, and still plays, a big role in our eating habits.

If the authorities were really open and honest about what people should eat, then they would have the food industry on their backs. This was a problem with most of the countries in the Western World.

Science and technology now made a vast difference in our food intake, and a new name for some of these were "Frankenstein Foods," simply because they had lost all relation to good, whole foods. Ingredients were ground, added to, tossed around in machines, and put back together to resemble foods, but in fact they were just a bundle of chemicals. How else do you think that a certain make of crisps can all turn out the same size and shape to fit into a cylinder?

The food market was becoming globalised and there was a political battle between the EU and the USA over standards and quality.

During this time, aspartame was being used world-wide. This is an artificial sweetener that seemed to be a good alternative to sugar. It became the answer to people's problems over sugar and soon, shelves were full of sugar-free foods, such as squash, yoghurts, chewing gum and candy.

Suspicions were aroused when this product first came out, but it was still produced as a healthy alternative to having sugary drinks and chewing gum. Dentists promoted sugar free gum, but are not doing that so much now that they, too, have become aware that aspartame is not the healthy product that it was originally promoted to be.

There is more research being done, but there is now evidence being shown that artificial sweeteners are actually making people fatter.

http://www.nbcnews.com/health/diet-fitness/how-can-diet-sodas-make-you-fat-study-may-explain-n205406

This decade brought with it an abundance of ready meals, and apparently the sales of ingredients for cooking went right down. If you looked for ingredients to make your own cake, it was hard to come by. The shelves were full of ready-made cakes or cake mixes.

Unfortunately, because of this, many children grew up never knowing how to cook. And now in the 2010's we are reaping the consequences. Many of today's adults don't even know how to boil an egg!

Then there were the salads. Even these were now ready-washed and prepared, thanks to a new packing technique. This would include ready-washed stir fries with a sauce in a sachet added to the package.

Snacks took on a whole new meaning. Where in years gone by, you took a biscuit out of a tin or packet, now the biscuit was a bar of something. Consequently, a snack increased from something like 80 calories with your coffee, to more like 200 or 300. Kellogg's' came up with the ingenious idea of inventing a cereal snack bar, and among them was a Special K snack bar, the cereal we discussed earlier.

Whilst the food industry was using people's concerns about their health, at the same time they were still selling Frankenstein foods. Whilst employing food "designers" to make food as addictive and tasty as possible in order to sell more, just down the aisle they were selling margarines that were purported to lower cholesterol and were therefore considered healthy. However, if you took the colour out of these margarines you would end up with a grey glob. Compare the list of ingredients in them to the ingredients in butter.

The cereal aisles were getting longer and longer, higher and higher, filling up with cereals that were toasted, flaked, sugar added, nuts and syrup added, dried fruit mixed in, even porridge with sugar added. Then there was a claim added to the packet that there were added vitamins, and that oats were healthy because they lowered your cholesterol (never mind the sugar.)

Geoffrey Bible, CEO in 1999 of Kraft, was interviewed by our friend Jacques Peretti, and he said that he warned the food industry that they were going the way of the tobacco industry, who had denied for many years that tobacco was not addictive and was not doing anyone any harm. He told them, "Be prepared to be fighting hard, when fighting hard is what's best for the business."

But the food industry responded by denying that this was the case.

So what was happening in the slimming world?

Diets that were around at this time were many. The internet was still relatively unused, and most diet books were in shops. By now, the slimming industry was having a boom-time. I have written a book reviewing 25 diets, and most of them were certainly around in the 90s, and they were only the most well-known.

Among them was the Atkins diet. Which was very similar to the Stillman diet mentioned in an earlier chapter. This was a very low-carbohydrate diet and high fat. It took the world by storm and although controversial, proved to be a big success. If you could stomach the large amounts of fat that were in this diet, then you seemed to be onto a winner.

Medical authorities were warning people against it, because it was still their belief that fat was the culprit in heart disease and obesity. It seemed to prove their point when Dr Atkins died suddenly. It was claimed that he died of a head injury after a fall. For years afterwards there were enquiries by the media into exactly what he did die of. We probably will never know. But this way of eating became a way that many people loved. And soon there were figures coming out to prove that their cholesterol and lipids in their bloodstream, had not gone up, which was the fear voiced by many experts.

The Paleo way of eating was also born, which is eating real food, but we will come to this when we look at the 2000's.

Out of this idea came the Zone diet, South Beach diet, and many other low carbohydrate diets.

Not too much had changed really in the pursuit of being slim from the 1890s to the 1990s.

People were still looking for the magic cure, and pills were still being sold with claims that they could make you lose weight.

There were and still are many supplements being sold purporting to do this. These claims are coming from many health food companies. Among the claims made are;

1. Green tea, chickweed and fennel will curb your cravings.

2. Guar gum and Physillium will make you feel full quicker.

3. Caffeine, Guarana, synphrine and B-complex vitamins will speed up your metabolism.

4. Green tea, hydrocitric acid and flax seed will slow down your body's fat production.

5. Chondritin will keep your body from absorbing fat.

Sorry folks, but none of these claims will help you very much, even if they are true, they will make very little difference. You will find the wording on most packets that goes something like, *"this will only work as part of a calorie controlled diet."* This is a cop out because if you are watching your calorie intake, you are eating a diet of healthy foods anyway; the supplement is not what is making the difference.

I am not saying that supplements are a waste of money per se, but that it is not a good idea to spend money on them specifically for weight loss.

It was in the latter years of this decade that a prescription pill was invented to block fat absorption.

Again, this sounded like a wonderful idea, until people encountered the side effects such as diarrhoea. The instructions told you that you still had to stick to a low fat diet, but people ignored that part and still thought that they could eat what they liked. Consequently the diarrhoea was so bad that they had to discontinue taking the pills.

So did things improve at the turn of the 21st century? Had people yet learned any more than they knew at the turn of the 20th century?

Chapter 11. 2000 to 2014: Diet Freedom? Or not?

The 21st Century on one hand is waking up to where we went wrong over the last 100 years, but on the other hand, there is a lot of controversy over fat, cholesterol, and carbohydrate.

The need for protein is not quite so questionable and neither is the amount. Protein is recognised as being absolutely essential for the human body to keep itself in good working order. It builds cells, rebuilds them when they are destroyed and maintains them.

The biggest controversy is the question of carbohydrate, as some experts are saying that you can actually live without it. I have written more about getting the balance right in my book *"Design Your Own Diet"* Amazon Kindle.

Carbohydrate is not the enemy that some make it out to be. The problems with this macronutrient are the amount and what foods you are obtaining it from.

Refined Carbohydrate is a no-no. This is food such as white flour and anything made with it, white rice, and any foods with added sugar. The body treats all three of these in the same way as sugar.

Here is a very simple explanation of how this works. When you eat sugar, your pancreas produces insulin, which in turn takes the sugar out of the bloodstream and stores it in fat cells. For a more detailed explanation of this process, look for the book, *Fat Chance* by Robert Lustig.

As for fat, at the time of this writing, January 2015, there are more and more reports coming out that saturated fat is not the enemy that it was originally thought to be.

So we can see that down through the ages, humans have changed their minds and their thinking over food and weight repeatedly.

Will we ever get it sorted?

In the late 70s and 80s and well into the 90s fat was the absolute enemy. Then, in the early 2000s people began to realise that there were certain fats that the body needed. Whereas in the 80s there were diets based on no or very little fat, now in the 21st century, we are being told that we must eat a certain amount of healthy fats.

In the early 21st century we were advised that healthy fats were olive oil, and other sun-pressed natural oils. We were still avoiding butter and saturated fats.

But now recently we are told that healthy fats include butter.

There are still people who are using the so-called healthy margarines. The way to tell a healthy fat or spread is to read the label. More than two ingredients are questionable. Some of these margarines take up the whole of the side of a pack with the list of ingredients, including colourings to make them look palatable.

One trend that has caught on is probiotics. Again, the food companies came along with their answer to probiotics, and produced little mini bottles with a liquid purported to contain probiotics. Folks, there are not enough of them by any stretch of the imagination in these little bottles. To get a healthy amount of these friendly bacteria, you need a good helping of natural bio-active yoghurt, without sugar and preferably not low fat. Add it to your own mix of muesli or fruit and you have a healthy, delicious meal.

In case you don't know what probiotics are, they are the millions of bacteria that live in a healthy gut and colon. They help your body to absorb the goodness from your food. A bad diet will destroy these little friends, as will a dose of antibiotics. So we need to eat a good, healthy diet and include probiotics in it. If you have been on a bad diet, or taken antibiotics, it is a good idea to take a course of probiotics in the form of tablets or capsules, and then keep them topped up with a healthy diet and a good helping of bio yoghurt every day.

Because the trend in the 21st century is beginning to grow away from unhealthy processed foods, farmer's markets and small shops are coming back into fashion. Here you will find mostly organic vegetables and local meats. The nearer your meat is grown from home, the healthier it will be. This is certainly the case in the UK, but I cannot speak for other countries.

Where in the three previous decades people were unaware of how their meat, poultry and fish were being reared, now we are becoming aware, and there is a definite move towards demanding that our meat is raised in a healthier way.

Hopefully, the day is approaching when the factory farming for all livestock will end. And it has to start with us as individuals.

I watched a film not so long ago about a huge consortium that has control over a lot of our food, and the farmers who grow and rear them. At the end they ask you to vote against these consortiums with your purse. It is the only way that we can beat them.

The importance of healthy dark greens is coming to the fore now too, and this is one thing that supermarkets are promoting. They are recognising the trend toward the importance of eating them.

The jury is still out on whole grains. They are certainly better for you than refined ones. But the main thing is that people are now more aware, and the fluffy white loaf of the 70s is fast disappearing. Not fast enough, but at least it is on the decline.

For many years, the chip pan was an important part of the household, but now people are moving towards oven chips.

A chip pan in the mid 1900s was a dangerous item in more ways than one. Firstly, the fat was used over and over again, thus becoming carcinogenic. Secondly, because it was an open pan heated on a hot plate, there was the danger of forgetting to switch it off, and the fat caught fire. Many emergency calls by the fire brigade were because someone had left the chip pan on!

It must be noted however, that there is becoming a split down the middle on food in the 21st century.

On the one hand, we have the move towards fresh and real organic foods, but on the other hand, we have the move to more takeaway and fast food outlets. In my local shopping area, consisting of all small shops, there is one butcher, two newsagents, two small supermarkets, a charity shop, a sun-tanning lounge, one small bank branch, a betting shop, a cash for your unwanted goods shop, a bakers, and seven different takeaways. How's that for a balanced community?

Many people claim that they cannot afford to eat healthily, yet the queues are often out across the pavement for these takeaways.

During the last couple of years, attention has been brought to the damage that sugar can do in the diet. So we are at last seeing a response now to the fact that people have become more prone to diseases such as obesity, heart disease, Type 2 Diabetes and stroke.

It may be worth pointing out at this point that nearly all processed foods have sugar in them. Read the label and you will be surprised. Even the cold meat at the deli counter has a sugar coating.

There is an odd phenomenon going on here. There is more attention coming to the damage that various foods can do, such as processed foods, refined, sugar, and un-healthy fats. Especially sugar. But when you sit in the waiting room and study the UK Eat Well plate, they are still saying that one third of your diet should consist of starchy foods. In fact, it is still stated "Base your meals on starchy foods!" The USA pyramid is a little better, but still not enough to make a difference.

So we have more and more people who are turning away from the unhealthy foods of the last three decades, but we have just as many, if not more, who still persist in eating unhealthily.

You cannot really blame people for being so confused. I bet in reading this you are a little confused, because there does not seem to be a clear guidance on what *HEALTHY* food is.

A very good way to find out is to look at anything that you can find about *The Paleo Diet*. Which is also often referred to as the primal way of eating. Roughly speaking,it bases itself on the hunter gatherer way of eating. Meat, fish, bird, eggs, nuts, berries, fruits in season, vegetables, leaves and seeds. This does not sound very much, but it actually encompasses a big variety of foods.

An interesting remark from a Jonathan G. F. Stowell in a report (link below) says that interest in healthy foods is increasing. This awareness is being created through the media, food manufacturers and *"to a lesser extent, by government health education programmes."* Isn't it remarkable that just after the Second World War the governments formed the WHO and yet they seem to be the last to change their minds and keep up with all the developments in healthy eating? I leave you to draw your own conclusions as to why that is.

Further on, Jonathan says *"Industry supports nutrition education in particular areas because it hopes to gain access to, or create, a profit opportunity. It invests money in an activity in the hope of eventual gain for the shareholders, and nutrition is no exception in that respect."*

http://www.euro.who.int/__data/assets/pdf_file/0005/96458/QU14598 EU.pdf

In the light of the fact that these diseases are increasing, I do wonder why the authorities just seem to be ignoring this. It is all very well to say that we must have five vegetables and fruits a day, but what they are omitting to say is that you need five a day of these foods to **replace** the other junk. Not on top of it!

To be fair though, it seems that the food industry can and does spend a large amount of money on research and the science of food, so perhaps that is one reason why the government tends to leave it to them.

I wonder how many of us are still in the mode of thought "It won't happen to me!"

The same mode of thought that says we can drive down the freeway or motor way too fast and believe ourselves invincible?

It is estimated that over the next thirty years, the number of people over the age of sixty will rise to nearly a quarter of the world's population.

A good amount of them will be the offspring of the Baby Boomers. Are we going to educate these people while they are in their 30s and 40s to see that they must look more carefully at their diet?

A lot is being said at this time about how it is reckoned that the offspring of today's grandmothers and grandfathers will not live as long as the older generation.

There are a good deal of Baby Boomers who are now in their 60s, who have fallen into bad eating habits, but there are just as many who do not take an interest in the modern processed and junk type foods that abound. If they are in any way to be shown to be not eating so well, it is usually due to too many biscuits and cake, rather than takeaways or fast foods.

Also, as discussed earlier in the chapter on the 1950s, many of them suffered malnutrition and this did not give them a good foundation for their older years.

Is it any wonder then, that there is such a lot of disease and obesity around in that generation? They are the ones who spent most of their adult years experiencing the changing trends in eating.

Firstly, they were on rations as kids, then they were let loose with the sudden increase in sweets, candy and sugary foods.

Followed by being told that they needed to not just cut down on fat, but to cut it out.

Then the development of processed, refined, junk, and fast foods and more and more takeaways.

And in the last twenty years or so, constant conflicting advice from the media about what is good and what is bad. Even scientists and people who are expert on the subject just cannot agree.

But for the sake of seeing the picture more clearly, let's compare this daily diet in from the 50s which I showed in chapter 5 to a typical daily diet of today.

1950's;

Breakfast would have been porridge, cornflakes toast and marmalade and sometimes an egg.

Lunch might have been sandwiches, meat paste or corned beef, or egg. Soup was popular for lunch times too. Salad would have consisted of lettuce, tomato, cucumber and maybe a little watercress. This was the time when salad cream, came into its own.

However, many working class people had the main meal of the day at lunch time (It would be known as dinner) and such meals as cottage pie, pasties, pies, steak and kidney pudding, sausage and mash and on Sunday, the proverbial roast. Chicken was a luxury and many had this for their Christmas dinner. Turkey was a rarity.

No home was complete without the jam, syrup, tomato sauce, brown sauce and mustard in the cupboard. Otherwise, there would be no other condiments, except if there as some pickle of some sort.

2015

Breakfast; A bowl of sugary cereal with skimmed milk, or a breakfast cereal bar.

Midmorning. A packet of crisps and/or a chocolate bar and a latte.

Lunch: A takeaway lunch of either a sandwich or sausage rolls. The sandwich could be anything between 350 calories for a healthy one with calories marked on it to a huge baguette with a heavy filling.

Or; Some sort of cooked takeaway such as southern fried chicken, fish and chips, curry and rice. Yesterday I was watching a worker in a local department store restaurant serving up curry and rice, and, as if that were not enough, there was a side of chips as well.

Followed by the latte coffee again and a cake or chocolate bar.

There may possibly be a piece of fruit, just as a token to make the meal feel healthy!

Mid-afternoon: When many people suffer from 4 o'clock low sugar syndrome. A doughnut or another chocolate bar. And a cup of tea or soda.

Evening: Could be a pizza or some other takeaway again. A ready meal. Or a cooked meal of some sort.

Bedtime. Must have a milky drink before I go to bed! Oh, and perhaps a sandwich. Or (yes, I have witnessed this) another takeaway. "I fancy a Chinese meal!" After a day of eating like this, is it any wonder that people have to resort to a slimming diet, such as the one below.

Something like this;

Breakfast; a slimming cereal such as Special K and skimmed milk.

Mid-morning: An apple or slimming cereal bar.

Lunch: Cold meat and salad with a "lite" calorie-counted dressing. Followed by a black coffee.

Mid-Afternoon; Same as mid-morning

Evening; A calorie-controlled, ready meal, or a salad, or a fat-free chunk of meat of some sort with vegetables and no fat used for the gravy. Followed by another piece of fruit.

No supper or a cup of tea with skimmed milk.

From that we can see that dieters go from one extreme to the other.

Do you want to know how I and a few of my Real Food friends eat?

Breakfast: Egg and bacon, mushrooms and tomatoes. Or yoghurt and home-made muesli.

Mid-morning: Nothing, because the good breakfast sustains them until lunchtime.

Lunch: A good helping of meat with salad and plenty of vegetables.

Mid-afternoon: Perhaps a cup of tea and a handful of nuts.

Evening: A really good helping of meat and vegetables again. Filling you up to satiation.

Followed by 2 or 4 squares of 85% chocolate.

A glass of red wine accompanies the evening meal a couple of times a week.

So back to the Baby Boomers then, they also have a better chance of remedying this. Firstly, because of the internet. There is lots of information about how you can improve your lifestyle, with good food, exercise, activities and how to eat better for your brain.

At the time of writing I am developing a new programme that will include all this.

It is not going to be like many other over-fifty websites with just the beauty and the well-known diet tips, but we'll be looking at how to change your thinking, what activities you can take part in, new careers, the real nutrition story, how to decide on medication, keeping you up to date with reports and expert opinions. A bit more of the nitty-gritty in other words.

It will be aimed at over sixty-five's as that is the general age for retirement and when people start to feel old! Not me, though! That is why I feel in a position to help.

We hear a lot about how people cannot afford to eat healthfully, don't we?

Well, I wonder what percentage of their income they actually spend on food.

My husband and I spend about £60 a week on food. This is what my weekly basket looks like.

Belly pork 4 slices, 4 lean pork chops, 500 grams of minced beef, a chicken or other joint of meat. 300 grams of cold turkey, a large cauliflower, a 2 kilo bag of potatoes, 1 large Swede, 4 or 5 large carrots, 3 onions, 7 large oranges, 10 bananas, 6 litres of whole milk, 400 grams of cheddar cheese, 200 grams of feta cheese, 2 bags of frozen berries, a cake or dessert of some sort for him (he likes something sweet in the evenings) 1 x500 gram pack of butter and 6 extra-large eggs.

Other occasional additions would be, porridge oats, oatmeal, dried pitted dates, bio-yoghurt (I make my own or buy depending on time, etc.) gravy mix, salt, pepper, herbs, tinned tomatoes, tinned tuna, cider vinegar, olive oil, garlic, and pickles. In my house, a bag of sugar is in the cupboard for about 6 months as it is only there for visitors. I use stevia, (lasts me about 6 months for a jar,) peanut butter (for the dogs) mustard, rice, pasta, frozen fish and meat.

Our meals consist of cooked porridge for hubby, and home-made muesli for me, at breakfast.

Salad or soup for me at lunchtime with either cheese or tuna followed by black coffee and 2 squares of 85% dark chocolate, sometimes a slice of German rye bread. Or if I am in a hurry or are particularly busy I will have a small helping of my muesli again.

A sandwich with 2 slices bread and cold meat and cucumber for him, followed by an orange and a banana.

Mid-afternoon I have an apple and sometimes a piece of feta cheese.

Evenings are either egg and bacon with tomatoes and baked beans, or meat and vegetables, perhaps a pizza for him if I am having an omelette; curry and rice, spaghetti Bolognese with rice for him and cauliflower for me.

Nothing after that, as I am quite full.

I use different recipes using herbs, spices, salt and pepper and garlic.

I look out for bargains of course, and buy them in when I see them.

Many people who would like to lose weight or keep a better eye on healthier foods, also use the excuse that home cooked foods and healthy foods are tasteless. But I for one can say that it is what you make it.

A slow cooker is a very useful item to have, not tucked away in the cupboard, but out in the open for use.

This will save you money and time. I often simply chuck in the meat; add seasoning and onions and maybe a few vegetables, and some water and a stock cube. Put it on first thing in the morning and get on with my day. Then when we come to eat in the evening all I have to do are a few vegetables which cook in 10 minutes and you have a delicious, nutritious meal. Which did not take any more time than putting a ready meal in the microwave, and it was certainly more nutritious and cheaper. Especially when cooking for the family.

You can do curries this way too, and eat them with rice.

People who are motivated to look after themselves and can see that it is important to look after their health, which includes being more healthy into their older years, or the third age, will do this and use no excuses.

Which category are you?

The ones who can't be bothered? Who are sick with no energy, and are always "coming down with something?"

Or are you among the ones who will decide to eat healthily, never have to worry about their weight, love themselves and appreciate what it is to have the energy to go for a walk, be out in the fresh air, and have a decent social life without the need to overindulge in too much food or alcohol and know that they can have just as good a time.

Nobody can guarantee that they will stay perfectly healthy for the rest of their life, no matter what they do. But if you have a healthy, nutritious diet, get plenty of exercise and fresh air, when you do have something wrong your body stands a better chance of fighting whatever it is.

Let's just take a look for a moment at someone who does not do this. For the sake of anonymity we will call him Bob. He is a single man, aged 48, and is a buyer in a small store.

Bob gets up in the morning and the first thing he does after using the bathroom, is light a cigarette and put the kettle on. He slings a piece of bread in the toaster, probably white and refined, looks out the window at the weather and thinks he would really rather stay at home. But he has got to go to work.

After showering, he eats the piece of toast slathered in butter and marmalade because it has gone cold and dry.

While stuck in a traffic jam, he is listening to the news and hears that the experts have changed their minds yet again over whether red wine is good for you or not. "I wish they'd make up their bloody minds!" he shouts at the radio.

On his arrival at work, the coffee machine is going and he always needs at least two cups to wake him up properly and get him in the mood for work. When the 11 o'clock break comes, the coffee machine has a box of doughnuts beside it. Even though he does not know who they belong to, he takes one anyway.

At 1 o'clock, the sandwich trolley comes around and he chooses cheese and pickle, a bag of crisps and healthy yoghurt to follow up. He also spies some salted peanuts, to keep on his desk in case he gets hungry again.

After eating his feast, it is time to return to work and he manages to keep going until 4pm this time. But by then he has got the shakes and is suffering from what he calls four o'clock low sugar. So he supposes that he ought to have something with sugar in to top him up. He is suffering from hypoglycemia. (Low blood sugar)

At the end of the day, some mates have invited him out for a drink. So even though he has to drive he thinks that one won't hurt and has a much longed-for beer. Then he jumps in the car and heads for home.

On the way, he feels hungry and tired and the thought of cooking something is just too much. So he decides that perhaps it will be a takeaway. Either pizza, Kentucky fried chicken or burger and chips perhaps. He actually eats this in the car, as he does not want it to go cold.

On reaching home at about 7.30 p.m., he changes out of his business clothes and into some shorts and a tee and settles down to watch some television with a beer straight from the fridge. Ah, that's the life! The next thing he knows, it is midnight. He has fallen asleep on the sofa and he is hungry again. So he grabs a packet of chips, or a snack of some kind, has another beer and drops into bed.

Spot the damage!

On the other hand, his mate Bill, who Bob thinks is a health freak, starts his day by cycling to work. He has already had a muesli and natural yoghurt for his breakfast.

On reaching work, he is wide awake and alert. He doesn't need the coffee to spur him on. He does not get hungry during the morning because the muesli has kept him going.

For lunch, he joins Bob at the sandwich cart, but he chooses the cold ham and salad sandwich. He has a yoghurt, but one of the plain ones, because there is no added sugar. He also chooses some smoked almonds and an apple.

At 4 p.m., he eats the almonds and has not had any low-sugar problems.

He joins Bob in the bar for a drink and chooses a red wine.

After cycling home, he changes and cooks himself a stir fry with chicken and rice noodles in a lovely black bean sauce. This is followed by a piece of fruit or maybe some strawberries and cream (Yes cream! He is not on a low-fat diet!)

He then does some work on his hobby, which is writing, as he is an author. Doing something creative rather than just wasting time.

At nine, he stops and decides it is time to chill out. He then has a healthy snack such as some more almonds or even a packet of peanuts.

He is not a health freak and the foods that he has eaten are not way out foods that normal people would not have. He has simply kept his eating under control because he has had very little sugar and starch.

Research shows that people are loathe to change their diets. They are not willing to sacrifice taste and texture for health.

But at the end of the day, even after 10,000 years, it seems that the human race has not yet sorted out the problem of overweight, and being fat. It does not seem to know what to do about it.

We discriminate; we call those who suffer, greedy, out of control, and even freaks. Yet there are more and more of us who are becoming overweight and increasing our chances of being obese.

There are billions of dollars and pounds poured into research for disease, medication for disease and treating it. Yet still we seem to persist in not paying enough attention to the evidence that eating too much of the wrong type of foods is making us ill.

We've looked at the way that scientists, authorities, and governments have ignored people who have shown evidence because it has not been proved. We seem to be going down a black hole at the mercy of powerful people who, like the fiasco over the tobacco crisis, are just claiming that eating the foods that are being dished up to people have nothing to do with the current health crisis.

Do you remember this from Chapter 2?

According to the medical dictionary found here; http://medical-dictionary.thefreedictionary.com/fad+diet

This is one definition of fad-diet.

"Any number of weight-reduction diets that either eliminate one or more of the essential food groups, or recommend consumption of one type of food in excess, at the expense of other foods. Fad diets rarely follow sound nutritional principles for weight loss, which focus on ingesting fewer calories and/or consuming more energy through exercise; fad diets are generally not endorsed by the medical profession."

However, here http://dictionary.reference.com/browse/fad

The reason why I said that I would discuss this definition further on is because this is the way that medical authorities are seeing a way of eating that is out of synch with what they believe is the right way.

They are simply dismissing the paleo or lower carbohydrate way of eating as fad dieting and putting many people off who could be benefitting from this way of eating.

I have discussed in this book ways that people have gone to the trouble to either avoid being fat, or lose it when they are.

In the chapter on the early 19th century we looked at the fad diets of the day. But a hundred years later, we are still doing the same. What happened to all those years of wasted research?

Young women are still dying of eating disorders such as anorexia. People abuse their bodies with purging after bingeing.

Obese people are now reaching gigantic measurements on the scales and hospitals are having to make special beds and wheelchairs to accommodate them. At this time the EU has brought legislation saying that obesity needs to be treated as a disability.

Disease and illnesses are on the increase. Type 2 Diabetes is getting out of control

Yet still the blame has been put on the individual.

What is needed is a fresh, new look at the problem. These days, with all the technology, science and research that can be done we have no excuse.

And yet, authorities, governments, the food industry, and we as individuals are just turning a blind eye.

Many of the reasons why the authorities are not doing as much as they should is because of their wallets!

The reason why individuals are not doing anything is because they feel helpless against the tide of conflicting advice and media reports.

So is it time to use the science, recognise that there is an answer, stop using excuses such as above, and look for yourself at what YOU can do as an individual?

If you have a weight or health problem yourself, can you look at your eating habits and change them?

Is it time to change your thinking and limiting beliefs!

Stop using the authorities and the food industry's indifference and do something about it yourself.

Do your own research and take some action!

Become aware of your own position in this.

Become aware of what you can do!

Epilogue

Right down through the centuries people have struggled with weight, except in the event of food shortages.

So what does this say? That of course we come back to the obvious. People who are obese or overweight have at some time eaten too much food. No matter whether you eat real food, junk food, processed food, vegetarian, vegan or raw food. If you eat more calories than your body needs, you will store fat. That is not because there is something wrong with you; it actually means that you are normal. Your body is doing what it was designed to do.

So what is the answer then?

1. Whatever size you are, accept yourself.

2. Love yourself.

3. Look at whether you are a size that is unhealthy and unattractive.

4. Make sure that it really is unattractive and not just because you think it is.

5. Stop comparing yourself to other people and get the criteria for this right.

6. Do not go on a restrictive calorie-counted diet.

7. Make sure that what you are eating is nutritious.

8. Make every single calorie you eat count!

9. Be aware that although you should not count calories, they do still exist!

10. Don't just go on the latest fad diet.

Have a look at my website for help to get it right for yourself, or for anyone you know who might value some help.

You can become a subscriber and sign up for the current FREE gift which varies from time to time.

There are details about my books, and other books that back up what I have said.

There are many blogs to check out.

My website is http:/www.patriciacherrylifecoach.com